T4-AJS-538

Assessment of
Performance Measures
for
Public Health, Substance Abuse,
and Mental Health

Edward B. Perrin and Jeffrey J. Koshel, *Editors*

Panel on Performance Measures and Data
for Public Health Performance Partnership Grants

Committee on National Statistics

Commission on Behavioral and Social Sciences and Education

National Research Council

NATIONAL ACADEMY PRESS
Washington, D.C.   1997

NATIONAL ACADEMY PRESS • 2101 Constitution Avenue, N.W. • Washington, D.C. 20418

NOTICE: The project that is the subject of this report was approved by the Governing Board of the National Research Council, whose members are drawn from the councils of the National Academy of Sciences, the National Academy of Engineering, and the Institute of Medicine. The members of the committee responsible for the report were chosen for their special competences and with regard for appropriate balance.

This report has been reviewed by a group other than the authors according to procedures approved by a Report Review Committee consisting of members of the National Academy of Sciences, the National Academy of Engineering, and the Institute of Medicine.

This study was supported by Contract No. 282-95-0034 between the National Academy of Sciences and the U.S. Department of Health and Human Services. Any opinions, findings, conclusions, or recommendations expressed in this publication are those of the author(s) and do not necessarily reflect the view of the organizations or agencies that provided support for this project.

Library of Congress Cataloging-in-Publication Data

Assessment of performance measures in public health, substance abuse, and mental health / Edward B. Perrin and Jeffrey J. Koshel, editors ; Panel on Performance Measures and Data for Public Health Performance Partnership Grants, Committee on National Statistics, Commission on Behavioral and Social Sciences and Education, National Research Council.
    p. cm.
   Includes bibliographical references (p.).
   ISBN 0-309-05796-5 (pbk.)
    1. Public health—Evaluation. 2. Public health—United States—Evaluation. I. Perrin, Edward. II. Koshel, Jeffrey. III. National Research Council (U.S.). Panel on Performance Measures and Data for Public Health Performance Partnership Grants.
RA427.A75 1997
362.1′0973—dc21

97-4915
CIP

Printed in the United States of America

iii

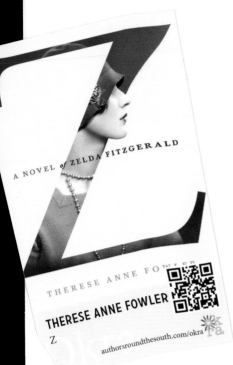

Contents

APPENDICES

Preface

In summer 1995, as part of its response to the need for assuring that public funding of health programs be related to documented program performance, the Office of the Assistant Secretary for Health of the U.S. Department of Health and Human Services (DHHS) requested that the National Research Council convene an expert panel to examine and report on the technical issues involved in establishing performance measures in ten substantive program areas. Such measures would be required as part of the proposed Performance Partnership Grants (PPG) Program, under which each state will negotiate with DHHS an action plan with performance objectives that are specific in terms of outcomes, processes, and capacity to be achieved over 3-5 years.

The panel divided its work into two phases. The objective of the first phase was a report to the Secretary of DHHS on performance measures in specified areas that would be useful to the PPG Program over the next 3-5 years. This report presents the panel's findings and recommendations of the first phase. In the second phase, the panel will consider and report on what needs to be done to improve performance measures, for example, by designing new data systems and surveys and increasing understanding of the relationship between programmatic interventions and health outcomes. This two-phase approach was adopted by the panel because of our conclusion that developmental work is needed in both the public and private sectors to adapt, refine, or add to existing data systems to make them more useful in performance measurement and to more clearly delineate the complex causal links between program processes and outcomes.

Because of the uncertainty about the structure of the substance abuse and mental health block grants legislation, as well as funding levels for various public health programs being considered for conversion to a PPG format, it is unlikely that PPG contracts between the federal government and state agencies will go into effect before fiscal 1998. Yet a growing number of states are moving to monitor and analyze outcomes on their own. Moreover, there appears to be a growing consensus within the public health, substance abuse, and mental health communities about the value of performance measurement. Indeed, many people believe that the case for increasing, or even maintaining, public funding will depend on documented program performance.

The development of performance measures is a continuation of earlier efforts to assess progress toward important public health goals. The broad acceptance of immunization rates and other such measures developed for Healthy People 2000, for example, has been instrumental in the creation of data bases and the mobilization of resources in many jurisdictions to assess progress toward those objectives.

The work of this panel has been furthered significantly by four regional meetings of state officials and consumers convened by DHHS—in Portland, Oregon; San Francisco, California; Chicago, Illinois; and Philadelphia, Pennsylvania—and by input from several national associations of state agency administrators (the National Association of State Alcohol and Drug Abuse Directors; the National Association of State Mental Health Program Directors; the Association of State and Territorial Health Officials; and the National Association of County and City Health Officials). DHHS stated that the purpose of the regional meetings was to "develop comprehensive lists of desired program results to initiate the process of developing performance objectives." Prior to the meetings, organizations representing potential PPG grant recipients were asked to consult on a state, regional, or national basis to solicit opinions from their membership about the PPG measures that are important for individual programs. Representatives of these institutional interests were invited to attend the regional meetings, and participants included representatives of state and local governments, public health groups, tribal governments, professional associations, providers, consumers, and advocacy groups. DHHS has actively involved these associations in soliciting information on potential measures and data sources for the PPG process.

Other efforts are under way to examine performance measures for areas of public health that are not included in the panel's charge. For example, two studies were recently completed at the Institute of Medicine (IOM), one focusing on community health performance measures and the other examining performance indicators, standards, and measures for accreditation and quality assurance for managed behavioral health care. The first study, conducted by the Committee on Using Performance Monitoring to Improve Community Health, developed prototypical sets of indicators for specific public health concerns that communities can use to monitor the performance of public health agencies, personal health care organizations, and other entities that can contribute to health improvement (Institute of Medicine, 1997b). The second study, conducted by the Committee on Quality Assurance and Accreditation Guidelines for Managed Behavioral Health Care, developed a framework for accreditation standards and quality improvements for managed behavioral health care and for developing, using, and evaluating performance indicators (Institute of Medicine, 1997c).

The panel is mindful of the great interest that surrounds the PPG concept: the eventual usefulness of our reports will depend on understanding and agreement by the federal and state officials and others who will be key players in implementing it. For that reason, this report was released in draft form for public comment. The panel was especially interested in receiving comments on its assessment of data availability and quality and the usefulness of the suggested measures in light of the limited empirical data that link program interventions to health outcomes. The panel received many comments, which contributed to this report; see Appendix D for an overview of the comments received and the panel's responses.

The panel appreciates the assistance of the staff of the Committee on National Statistics (CNSTAT) in preparing this report: Miron Straf, staff director of CNSTAT for developing the original project design; Telissia Thompson for organizing panel meetings; Anu Pemmarazu for preparing key technical materials; Theresa Raphael for preparing the literature review for the panel and preparing the annotated bibliography; and Michelle Ruddick and Ashley Bowers for coding and analyzing the responses from the field. Thanks also go to Sue Skillman, University of Washington, for her valued assistance to the committee chair. Finally, special thanks go to Jeff Koshel, study director for this panel, for his very capable management of the study process.

Edward Perrin, *Chair*
Panel on Performance Measures and Data for
Public Health Performance Partnership Grants

The National Academy of Sciences is a private, nonprofit, self-perpetuating society of distinguished scholars engaged in scientific and engineering research, dedicated to the furtherance of science and technology and to their use for the general welfare. Upon the authority of the charter granted to it by the Congress in 1863, the Academy has a mandate that requires it to advise the federal government on scientific and technical matters. Dr. Bruce M. Alberts is president of the National Academy of Sciences.

The National Academy of Engineering was established in 1964, under the charter of the National Academy of Sciences, as a parallel organization of outstanding engineers. It is autonomous in its administration and in the selection of its members, sharing with the National Academy of Sciences the responsibility for advising the federal government. The National Academy of Engineering also sponsors engineering programs aimed at meeting national needs, encourages education and research, and recognizes the superior achievements of engineers. Dr. William A. Wulf is president of the National Academy of Engineering.

The Institute of Medicine was established in 1970 by the National Academy of Sciences to secure the services of eminent members of appropriate professions in the examination of policy matters pertaining to the health of the public. The Institute acts under the responsibility given to the National Academy of Sciences by its congressional charter to be an adviser to the federal government and, upon its own initiative, to identify issues of medical care, research, and education. Dr. Kenneth I. Shine is president of the Institute of Medicine.

The National Research Council was organized by the National Academy of Sciences in 1916 to associate the broad community of science and technology with the Academy's purposes of furthering knowledge and advising the federal government. Functioning in accordance with general policies determined by the Academy, the Council has become the principal operating agency of both the National Academy of Sciences and the National Academy of Engineering in providing services to the government, the public, and the scientific and engineering communities. The Council is administered jointly by both Academies and the Institute of Medicine. Dr. Bruce M. Alberts and Dr. William A. Wulf are chairman and vice chairman, respectively, of the National Research Council.

Assessment of
Performance Measures
for
Public Health, Substance Abuse, and Mental Health

Executive Summary

The Panel on Performance Measures and Data for Public Health Performance Partnership Grants was established at the request of the U.S. Department of Health and Human Services (DHHS). Its charge is to examine the state of the art in performance measurement for public health and to recommend measures that could be used to monitor the Performance Partnership Grant agreements to be negotiated between each state and the federal government. The panel was asked to consider performance measures in ten areas, which are clearly a subset of the full range of traditional public health concerns: chronic diseases; sexually transmitted diseases (STDs), human immunodeficiency virus (HIV) infection, and tuberculosis; mental health; immunization; substance abuse; and three areas of prevention of special interest to DHHS—sexual assault, disabilities, and emergency medical services. This report focuses on measures that states and the federal government can use over the next 3 to 5 years to negotiate agreements and monitor performance in these areas. A later report will examine additional measures that might be developed from new research findings on program effectiveness or as improvements are made to state and federal surveys and data systems.

More than 3,200 measures were proposed to the panel through various outreach efforts. The panel used four guidelines for assessing them: (1) the measure should be specific and result oriented; (2) the measure should be meaningful and understandable; (3) data should be adequate to support the measure; (4) the measure should be valid, reliable, and responsive. The measures that scored the highest are those we recommend for use in performance monitoring. They cover health status, social functioning, consumer satisfaction, and risk status.

In assessing the adequacy of data for specific performance measures, the panel concluded that there are few available data sources that are ideal for performance monitoring. Understanding the limits of available data is important if appropriate inferences are to be drawn. Many federal efforts to collect health-related data, for example, provide national rates, but do not collect data that provide state-level rates. Even when data are available at the state level, if comparisons are to be made among states, attention must be paid to the effect of different data collection methods on the comparability of results. Other issues that need to be considered include whether or not specific populations of interest are included in samples from which data are drawn and whether data are collected sufficiently often, or are made available soon enough, to be useful in the monitoring process.

It is important to note that many of the performance measures presented in this report can, and should, be subdivided to focus on specific high-risk populations in a state. These populations may be defined demographically, such as minorities, children, or elderly persons; by conditions, such as not having health insurance or being homeless; or by geographic area, such as central cities, high-risk neighborhoods, or rural communities. Specific subpopulations of interest vary across states. Rather than create multiple submeasures for each proposed measure, the panel chose, in most cases, to identify broad population measures that can be tailored by each state to focus on its specific population group priorities.

Despite their widespread use and intuitive appeal, health outcome measures are insufficient by themselves for monitoring the efforts of a given program in reducing complex public health problems. Many measures that are recognized as valid for tracking health outcomes are affected by many factors (inputs or processes), so changes in outcomes cannot be attributed only to specific program effectiveness. Attribution of responsibility for outcomes becomes even more difficult when the services in question are supported by multiple funding sources or multiple provider organizations. The panel concludes that performance monitoring must make use of process and capacity measures to complement available measures of outcomes. The panel recommends that each process and capacity measure be accompanied by reference to published clinical guidelines or other professional standards that describe the relationship between the process measure or capacity measure and the desired health outcome.

Given the current and potential uses of performance measurement in public health, substance abuse, and mental health, the panel recommends that a combination of measures of health outcome, process, and capacity be used in the agreements between the federal government and states. Because in some cases actual health status outcomes are impractical to measure or because there are many factors that affect the ultimate health outcome, the panel recommends using "intermediate" outcome measures, such as risk status, for which there is general consensus that the result being measured is related to the health status outcome. The panel uses the following definitions in this report:

Health Outcome: Change (or lack of change) in the health of a defined population related to an intervention, characterized in the following ways:

health status outcome:	change (or lack of) in physical or mental status
social functioning:	change (or lack of) in the ability of an individual to function in society
consumer satisfaction:	response of an individual to services received from health provider or program

Risk Status (intermediate outcome): Change (or lack of) in the risk demonstrated or assumed to be associated with health status.

Process: What is done to, for, with, or by defined individuals or groups as part of the delivery of services, such as performing a test or procedure or offering an educational service.

Capacity: The ability to provide specific services, such as clinical screening and disease surveillance, made possible by the maintenance of the basic infrastructure of the public health system, as well as by specific program resources.

Because of data limitations and differing health and defined population priorities among states, the panel's list of health outcome measures should be considered an important subset, but not an exhaustive listing, of those that will be of interest to state agencies around the country. Few states have adequate data to support every health outcome measure, and virtually all states have major priorities in addition to the ones indicated by these particular measures. Similarly, for process and capacity measures, there are many reasonable strategies that states can pursue to improve health outcomes, and each strategy requires a different set of process and capacity measures. Therefore, the panel offers representative examples of relevant process and capacity measures in each program area.

The potential health outcomes and risk status measures to be used for monitoring purposes are presented in Chapter 3 and described in detail in Appendix C. For each health topic covered, the report includes examples of process and capacity measures that complement the outcome and risk status measures suggested by the panel. Potential measures for chronic disease focus on improvement of health risk status for tobacco use, nutrition, exercise, and clinical screenings. For STDs, HIV infection, and tuberculosis, the potential outcome measures target reporting of incidence and prevalence rates for specific diseases; client satisfaction with treatment, and reduction of high-risk behavior among specific subpopulations at high risk of contracting or spreading the diseases. The immunization measures include a set for monitoring the incidence of vaccine-preventable disease and a set to be used to track vaccination rates for specific diseases. Most of the potential mental health measures focus on health outcomes for the treated population. Lack of data for measures of mental health outcomes in more general populations severely limits the number of potential measures the panel proposes. In substance abuse, the potential measures cover both treated and general populations for health status outcome, social functioning outcome, and risk status. For the three areas of prevention—sexual assault, disabilities, and emergency medical services—the narrowness of this charge to the panel and the general dearth of supporting data have resulted in a short list of potential measures.

Of course, use of even a large number of health outcome, process, and capacity measures may still result in less than conclusive evidence of agency or program performance in reducing multifaceted health problems. Therefore, the panel recommends that public health performance measures be considered as a central but not the only element of a continuous program of technical assistance. For example, if one measure or a combination of measures suggests that a given state is having unusual difficulty in making progress in meeting its performance objectives, such information should trigger an alert that some additional resources or technical assistance may be needed. The panel believes that this approach is consistent with the National Performance Review initiative at the federal level and with the total quality management activities that are being undertaken by state and local agencies around the country.

A major goal of this report is to provide an analytic framework for states and DHHS to use when assessing the appropriateness of specific outcome, process, and capacity measures for individual performance agreements. Recognizing that data resources and measurement methods need improvement, the panel recommends that DHHS continue to work with states toward several infrastructure goals: developing common definitions and measurement methods; encouraging efficient development of data resources that support multiple public health, mental health, and substance abuse needs; incorporating state data priorities in national infrastructure development efforts; and promoting states' data collection and analytic capabilities.

During the next stage of the study, the panel will examine the adequacy of existing databases to support improved health outcome measures, assess the quality of the empirical evidence of the effectiveness of specific interventions and the health outcomes discussed in this report, and suggest modifications to existing data sources or new databases necessary to support refined or new performance measures. Based on that assessment, the panel will recommend priority areas of research and data collection and infrastructure development for each of the health areas covered in this report, as well as for more general areas of public health concern.

1

Introduction and Framework

BACKGROUND

At the request of the U.S. Department of Health and Human Services (DHHS), the panel is assessing the state of the art for performance measures for public health programs. The goal is to recommend a set of measures for use by local, state, and federal officials to assist in evaluating progress toward public health goals. Such measures would be an integral part of Performance Partnership Grant (PPG) arrangements between a state and the federal government. Under a negotiated PPG agreement, as currently proposed, DHHS and each state would agree on a set of objectives and performance measures for individual federal-state grants; see box for definitions. These agreements will identify specific outcomes, processes, and capacity objectives for a period of 3-5 years. The PPG program will offer states increased control over funding priorities and program management of certain categorical programs in return for accepting increased accountability for results.

Performance Measure: a quantitative indicator that can be used to track progress toward an objective, i.e., to detect change over time and difference in change across programs

Objective: a specific level of measurable attainment between two points in time

In addition to the interest of DHHS and some members of Congress in applying performance measures to public health programs, several other factors seem to account for the growing interest in performance measurement systems. Such systems promise improved documentation of the achievements of public and private agencies and also serve to identify areas needing improvement. In fact, many people in public health believe that funding cannot be expected to increase or even be maintained at current levels without better documentation of the return on program investments. Performance measurement can also complement and extend on-going public health monitoring efforts, including Healthy Cities, Healthy Communities, and Healthy People 2000 and 2010, as well as state benchmarking activities and state efforts to develop systems to monitor managed care providers. Finally, the Government Performance and Results Act (GPRA) requires the federal government to measure the performance of all federal programs. As a result, some administrators of health programs at the federal, state, and local levels are concerned that the implementation process for the GPRA may become dominated by concerns of fiscal management unless good public health measures are available to evaluate program effectiveness.

As articulated by DHHS, the PPG concept envisions that DHHS, in consultation with states, public health professionals, private organizations, public agencies, and citizens, will develop a broad menu of performance measures that can be used in one or more of the following ten areas: chronic diseases; sexually transmitted diseases (STDs), human immunodeficiency virus (HIV) infection, and tuberculosis; mental health; immunization; substance abuse; and three subcategories of prevention of special interest to DHHS—sexual assault, disabilities, and emergency medical services. Each state-federal PPG agreement would specify performance measures as a basis for monitoring the program objectives selected for that state. DHHS has proposed that a small set of measures be designated as "core" measures of health problems or opportunities of national importance. Although these core measures would be monitored in each state, not all states would necessarily be required to address them as program priorities, since not every problem of national importance is a problem or priority in every state. A key element of the PPG concept is that progress toward the programmatic objectives is monitored through data regularly reported by the state.

To assist DHHS in developing the plan for the PPG program, the panel was charged with the following tasks: (1) to identify measurable objectives that states and other interested parties might want to achieve through PPG agreements that can be monitored at the state and national level, either now or with small modifications to existing data systems; (2) to identify measures relevant to PPG agreements that cannot be assessed but that are important to states and the federal government and therefore require further development; and (3) to recommend improvements to state and federal surveys and data systems to facilitate future collection of information for both existing and developmental measures. Task 1 is the subject of this report; tasks 2 and 3 will be the subject of a subsequent report. In carrying out tasks 2 and 3, the panel will pay careful attention to data adequacy and assess the need for additional data sources and program effectiveness research to supplement those that are currently available.

Candidate PPG measures that were assessed by the panel came from attendees at four regional meetings—more than 1,500 people—sponsored by DHHS during late 1995 and early 1996 and from professional associations. More than 3,200 candidate PPG measures were proposed to the panel.

STUDY FRAMEWORK

The panel views its role as a technical one, to identify and assess measures that states can use to evaluate their progress toward important health objectives and to recommend actions to improve the utility of such measures. This report provides an assessment of measures that could be used over the next 3-5 years by states and the federal government to monitor progress in meeting agreed-upon health objectives. The report does not attempt to review all of the program options and policies to be considered in structuring PPG agreements between DHHS and states: such issues as funding levels, matching requirements, hold-harmless funding provisions, allocation of resources decisions, financial incentives, and the like are not covered. The panel's goal is to provide technically sound methods for assessing progress in meeting public health objectives and to provide states and others with practical and useful tools to advance their public health objectives.

The panel's framework for assessing potential performance measures is simple: a public health program operating at the state level, with a certain size and structure (capacity), uses the resources provided by a federal funding program (process) to improve the health of the population it serves. The panel assumes that the effectiveness of a state program in using resources can most appropriately be evaluated by assessing the degree to which desired changes in health outcomes are achieved, together with a judgment of the degree to which those changes can be attributed to a program. When a firm causal link between the resources and processes used and the health outcome sought has not been established, as is often the case, or when the program resources are a small part of all the resources that contribute to the outcome, the panel believes that performance assessment must necessarily depend on a combination of health outcome, process, and program capacity measures. Furthermore, the panel suggests that performance measures be understood and adopted as the product of an evolutionary process, to be revised as additional empirical evidence is obtained and better methods of data collection are implemented.

DEFINITIONS

Public Health

In considering performance measures for public health programs, the panel was mindful of the concept of "core" public health functions developed by the Institute of Medicine (IOM) that is now widely accepted within the public health community. These core functions are assessment, policy development, and assurance (Institute of Medicine, 1988); see box. The IOM report also states that public health programs should include both disease prevention and health promotion, with "health" encompassing physical, mental, and environmental health.

The ten specific areas that the panel was asked by DHHS to examine with regard to performance measures are a subset of the full range of public health concerns. Many critical responsibilities of state and local public health agencies, such as maternal and child health, injury prevention, and environmental health, are not covered in this report, but the guidelines for assessing performance measures presented here can be applied to these other areas.

It is important to note that state public health departments are not always the designated recipients of federal funds. In the areas of substance abuse and mental health, for example, the grantee may well be the state department of human services. In many states, public health responsibilities are distributed among local districts. A PPG agreement in any given state, therefore, will need to clearly identify lines of responsibility and assure that the performance goals are reasonable given the organzational structure and resources available.

Public Health Assessment: "the regular and systematic collection, assembly, analysis and dissemination of information on the health of the community. This information includes statistics on health status, community health needs, and epidemiologic and other studies of health problems."

Public Health Policy Development: "the development of comprehensive public health policies by promoting use of the scientific knowledge base in decision-making about public health and by leading in developing public health policy."

Public Health Assurance: "assures that services necessary to achieve agreed upon goals are provided, either by encouraging actions by other entities (private or public sector), by requiring such actions through regulation, or by providing services directly" (Institute of Medicine, 1988:7-8).

Health Outcome: Change (or lack of change) in the health of a defined population related to an intervention, characterized in the following ways:

    health status outcome: change (or lack of) in physical or mental status
    social functioning: change (or lack of) in the ability of an individual to function in society
    consumer satisfaction: response of an individual to services received from health provider or program

Risk Status (intermediate outcome): Change (or lack of) in the risk demonstrated or assumed to be associated with health status.

Process: What is done to, for, with, or by defined individuals or groups as part of the delivery of services, such as performing a test or procedure or offering an educational service.

Capacity: The ability to provide specific services, such as clinical screening and disease surveillance, made possible by the maintenance of the basic infrastructure of the public health system, as well as by specific program resources.

Outcomes, Risk Status, Process, and Capacity

Health outcome, risk status, process, and capacity measures are all needed at different times and in different situations to intelligently monitor both changes in the health status of defined populations and the performance of all public and private agencies in working toward specified health goals; see box for definitions adopted by the panel for this report. In some cases, actual health outcomes are impractical to measure as indicators of program performance because too much time is required between intervention and outcome or because many confounding factors affect the ultimate health outcome. In such cases, the panel recommends using an "intermediate" measure, risk status, for which there is general consensus that the result being measured is related to the health outcome.[1]

Meaningful analysis of performance requires determining whether desired health outcomes are achieved, whether specific agency committments are carried out, and whether the agency has the capacity to conduct all the necessary processes. Outcomes are fundamental, and any process or capacity measure used to

---

[1]Although many of the "risk status" outcome measures in this report might otherwise be considered "process" measures, classifying such measures as "intermediate" outcomes is more appropriate in view of the short-term nature of the proposed performance agreements.

assess performance should be widely accepted as closely related to them. For example, if a state's PPG goal is to reduce its mortality rate from breast cancer, it can reduce the risk of such an adverse health outcome by increasing the number of mammograms it provides to women aged 50 and over. However, there are also a series of process activities (e.g., health education programs, requirements that private insurers include coverage of, say, mammography, surgical and nonsurgical treatment, and postoperative follow-up care) and capacity indicators (e.g., number of trained staff and facilities offering mammography screening) that are believed to be related to the level of mortality from breast cancer and can be monitored over time. A detailed set of such measures could provide some understanding of what particular service mechanisms are present and may affect the trend in the outcomes of interest. The capacity of public agencies is important for any comprehensive and accurate assessment of program performance. Infrastructure activities, such as the maintenance of various public health data and surveillance systems, are as important as monitoring drinking water quality and conducting restaurant inspections in promoting the public health. The panel notes, in fact, that DHHS supported a major study of public health infrastructure, which is expected to provide infrastructure capacity measures for use in the PPG process (Lewin-VHI, Inc., 1997).

ASSESSMENT GUIDELINES

In considering how to assess the appropriateness of individual measures for tracking the performance of state public health agencies under the PPG process, the panel reviewed materials developed by DHHS, state partners, and other professional groups (see Annotated Bibliography). The panel established guidelines for the assessment of proposed measures:

1. Measures should be aimed at a specific objective and be result oriented. PPG measures must clearly specify a desired public health result, including identifying the population affected and the time frame involved. Process and capacity measures should clearly specify the health outcome, or long-term objective, to which they are thought to be related.

2. Measures should be meaningful and understandable. Performance measures must be seen as important to both the general public and policy makers at all levels of government and they should be stated in nontechnical terms.

3. Data should be adequate to support the measure. Adequate data on the populations of interest must be available for the use of measures and have the following characteristics:

• Data to track any objective must meet reasonable statistical standards for accuracy and completeness;

- Data to track any objective must be available in a timely fashion, at appropriate periodicity, and at reasonable cost; and
- Data applied to a specific measure must be collected using similar methods and with a common definition throughout the population of interest. Comparisons of a measure across states are valid only if the definition and collection methodology are consistent across states.

4. Measures should be valid, reliable, and responsive. Measures should, as much as possible, capture the essence of what they purport to measure (i.e., be unbiased and valid for their intended purpose), be reproducible (i.e., reliable), and be able to detect movement toward a desired objective (i.e., be responsive).

That a measure can be valid for one purpose but not for another is an important factor in performance measurement. For example, a state's infant mortality rate is usually considered a valid measure in assessing the actual change in a state's rate of infant death from one period to another, but changes in that rate may not be a valid measure of the performance of an individual public health agency: the agency may have no control over many factors that can affect infant mortality, such as changing socioeconomic conditions or the demographic characteristics of the population. Performance measures must also be reliable: have a high likelihood of yielding the same results on repeated trials and, therefore, low levels of random error in measurement. Similarly, performance measures should be known to be responsive to change at the level of change that one would like to detect.

In an ideal world, each performance measure would fully satisfy all four guidelines; unfortunately, not many available health outcome measures can do so. For example, many factors not under a state agency's control can affect health outcomes, compromising the validity of measures of program effect. Consequently, the panel recommends that health outcome measures be used in conjunction with process and capacity measures to derive appropriately conservative inferences about the performance of a state agency. This approach will provide public officials and consumers with an opportunity to examine steps taken by agencies to achieve specific health outcomes and to better understand whether changes in the magnitude or direction of particular strategies should be considered. A combination of health outcome, process, and capacity measures should be used to identify what additional research is needed to establish more precisely the relations among program interventions and outcomes.

It is important that agencies that engage in performance monitoring specify the assumed relationship between any process or capacity measure proposed and the particular health outcome to which it is believed to be related and document, with empirical evidence and professional judgment, the assumed relationship. If states elect to implement new, experimental approaches to realize PPG objectives, they must collect the data necessary to document the effectiveness of those interventions.

One of the constraints of the PPG process, as currently formulated, is that the performance objectives must be judged capable of realization within 5 years. Yet many important public health objectives, such as lowered incidence of cancer and HIV infection, cannot be achieved over this short time period. However, it would be unwise to divert resources from those objectives simply because demonstrable results cannot be expected in the 5-year period. The panel recommends that DHHS and the states consider negotiating some items in their performance agreements that allow for longer term goals if relevant risk behaviors and process data can be used to measure progress toward the desired health outcomes.

2

Current Data Sources that Can Support PPG Measures

When a measure is proposed for use in PPG monitoring, appropriate data must be available to support its use. Unfortunately, few data sources are ideal for this purpose.

Although many types of data that have some applicability to monitoring the health of state populations are collected and assembled across the country, few come from concerted efforts to monitor the effects of public health interventions. In an ideal situation, data would be collected from the specific population of interest (or a representative sample); within the relevant time frame; using valid, reliable, and responsive measures. However, collecting and assembling data are expensive, and expanding data collection efforts can reduce the resources available for programs. As a result, the PPG process will often have to rely on data collected for one purpose or for generalized purposes to address another purpose, and states and the federal government must understand limitations of the applicability of the data. For example, the Centers for Disease Control and Prevention (CDC) supports the National Notifiable Diseases Surveillance System (NNDSS), which is designed to monitor, on a weekly basis, the occurrence of a set of diseases important to public health (including diphtheria, hepatitis A and B, STDs, tuberculosis). The NNDSS receives reports from all 50 states, five U.S. territories, New York City, and Washington, D.C., but it was designed primarily to identify outbreaks of specific diseases for rapid public health intervention, not to calculate precise incidence or prevalence rates across the country. Not all cases of the diseases receive medical care (which is how reporting usually originates), not all conditions are accurately diagnosed, not all diagnosed conditions are reported, and the completeness of reporting varies among participants.

NNDSS data might provide a gross measure of a state's changing rate of a reported disease, but not be appropriate (except for a few diseases) for comparing small changes in rates of incidence.

The lack of appropriate data may be the most important factor limiting effective monitoring of public health performance. States and the federal government may need to use data collected for other purposes and to rely on data that are not entirely comparable across states. Understanding the limits of such data is important if performance monitoring is to be effective.

One use of public health performance measures might be to examine and compare the effects of public health interventions among states. In that case, individual states and the federal government will want to compare the outcomes of similar (and different) interventions in different settings. For this purpose, comparable health outcomes data are needed from all states. However, states have had little incentive to standardize their data collection efforts with those of other states. A notable exception has been the development of the vital statistics system, a cooperative state-federal administrative data system that contains considerable health information. Data collection efforts at the national level (sponsored by the federal government or organizations with national and multistate agendas) are usually in a better position to collect health-related data using comparable definitions, questions, and methods across many or all states. Others, such as the Behavioral Risk Factor Surveillance System (BRFSS) and the Health-care Cost and Utilization Project, use similar questions and definitions but differ in methods. Largely because of budget constraints, however, national data collection efforts such as the National Health Interview Survey (NHIS) usually have as their objective the provision of national population estimates of health, and they have not yet had the sample size or sample design required to make state-level estimates.

Two surveys designed to generate state-level estimates are the National Immunization Survey (NIS) and the BRFSS. The NIS is a random-digit-dial telephone survey of households with small children, using samples drawn from all 50 states, Washington, D.C., and 27 metropolitan areas. The survey yields state and regional estimates of immunization completeness for children aged 19-35 months. This federally run survey uses comparable data collection methods across all states and regions, and comparisons of rates of immunization can reasonably be made among states.

BRFSS is a state survey designed to assess the prevalence of health-related behavioral risk factors associated with the leading causes of premature death and disability. It is a random-digit-dial survey of samples that can be generalized to state populations. While the CDC provides overall support and technical oversight for the BRFSS, individual states administer the survey and have the opportunity to add their own questions. As a result, sampling design and data collection methods may vary from state to state. Consequently, BRFSS data should be used cautiously when making comparisons among states. For example, if states have significantly different BRFSS response rates, users of the data should consider how nonresponse bias may have affected estimates of differences among the state rates being compared.

Other differences in data collection methods that affect data comparability are mode of collection (e.g., substance abuse rates ascertained from mail surveys or computer-aided interviews may be more accurate than those from telephone or in-person interviews) and use of proxy respondents (e.g., rates of breast self-examination may be more accurate if proxy responses are not allowed). Lack of complete comparability does not preclude using different data sources when making comparisons among states or populations, but the limits to comparability need to be considered when drawing conclusions about observed differences. Data comparability is also an issue, of course, when examining changes over time within a state. The effects of changes as well as state-to-state differences in data collection and analysis methods should always be of concern to data users.

In spite of its limitations for making comparisons among states, BRFSS (as well as a variety of other state-operated population surveys) may be a more convenient model than other federally directed surveys for assessing a state's progress toward meeting some PPG performance goals. States have considerable flexibility to add their own questions to this ongoing survey, and new questions do not require the same level of review required by law and regulation of many national surveys. In addition, because the sampling procedures and survey mechanism are established and ongoing, adding questions is relatively inexpensive.

Some data sources provide state-level data for some, but not all, states. For example, with CDC support, 49 states and Washington, D.C., have or are planning statewide tumor registries that capture incidence rates for most cancers. Other national efforts to collect health-related data from all states are often incomplete because they rely on voluntary state submission of the data. In these cases, such as with the National Facility Register of Substance Abuse Treatment and Prevention Programs, state data are often effectively not available because of long lag times in their submission.

Some regional, national, and other population-specific sources may be useful in PPG monitoring even if they do not provide state-level data. If a state adopts a PPG goal of increasing influenza vaccination rates among the elderly residents of a major metropolitan area, for example, it would be necessary to have data to measure progress toward that goal. The NHIS includes samples of specific large metropolitan areas in the United States and could be a source of data for such a measure. Data from a range of metropolitan areas surveyed through the NHIS might help to distinguish changes attributable to state interventions from changes that reflect national trends. National data that might serve as useful comparisons for monitoring changes in measures of the health status of state populations include the NHIS, the Medical Expenditure Panel Survey, Monitoring the Future, the National Hospital Discharge Survey, and the Healthcare Cost and Utilization Project. These national-level data may also be useful in distinguishing changes in rates specific to a state from those resulting from more general changes in the national environment. However, users need to consider comparability issues for these sources, too. Data may be collected at state or substate levels with different methods than those used to collect the national-level data. As noted above, for example, because each state's BRFSS survey is conducted independently and because response rates vary by state, BRFSS data cannot confidently be aggregated across all 50 states to obtain national-level estimates.

Another source of data that may be of potential use in PPG monitoring is the Drug Abuse Warning Network (DAWN). Although DAWN does not provide state-level rates, it does provide estimates of the number of drug-related visits to hospital emergency departments in 21 metropolitan areas of the country and of the number of drug-related deaths in 40 metropolitan areas. If a state targets reduction in emergency room admissions due to alcohol and other drug abuse as one of its performance objectives, monitoring that rate within a major metropolitan area may be an appropriate and practical measure of performance, especially if data are not available from elsewhere in the state. The state should consider how the metropolitan population represents the population of interest and whether any confounding factors might influence the data, such as availability and use of hospitals run by the Indian Health Service or the Department of Veterans Affairs, which are not included in the DAWN surveillance system.

Other state data sources may be useful in PPG monitoring, such as the hospital discharge data system maintained in many states (e.g., the CHARS data system in the state of Washington). Some states conduct their own population surveys to assess health status and insurance coverage. Trauma registries are maintained by many states, and Medicaid claims files are available in various forms in many states. Of course, if these data are to be used for PPG purposes, comparisons across states will be valid only if the relevant data are collected comparably and cover comparable populations and the inferences are not extended beyond specific subpopulations (e.g., Medicaid patients).

Frequency of collection and turnaround time are important considerations when assessing the utility of any data source in PPG monitoring. If performance measures are designed to detect changes in 3-5 years, at least two data collection points must be in the time frame of interest, and the data must be available for analysis within a reasonable time after collection. Many potential data sources for PPG monitoring may not be useful because slow turnaround times make them inaccessible in the required time frames or because policy decisions or budget constraints delay or halt continuing data collection.

Appendix B summarizes currently available data sources for health-related data that may be useful in PPG monitoring. The table indicates whether the source provides data at the national or state level and whether it provides data for all or some states, as well as the general type of data and the frequency of collection in each case.

As partnerships between the states and federal government are established through the PPG mechanism, interest in improving data sources for monitoring PPGs will probably increase. This state-federal collaboration (as well as state-local collaboration) offers great potential for identifying and finding methods to collect the most useful data for PPG monitoring. Identifying methods to improve data resources for PPG monitoring will be a major component of the second phase of the panel's work.

3

Potential PPG Measures for 1997–2002

To facilitate the review of the hundreds of candidate performance measures discussed at the regional meetings and provided to the panel, the panel divided into working groups corresponding to the health areas within its purview. Each working group followed the same general procedure for reviewing the candidate measures (using the measure assessment guidelines described in Chapter 1):

1. classify all of the proposed measures using the framework developed by the full panel;
2. select measures that appear to be clear and measurable;
3. review and select measures remaining after step 2. for adequacy of data source(s);
4. review and select measures remaining after step 3. for validity, reliability, and responsiveness;
5. select from the remaining outcome measures[1] those that can provide valid assessment of actions that might be taken at the state level within 3-5 years;
6. select examples of relevant process and capacity measures for each health area (see discussion below).

Many of the performance measures discussed below can and should be used

---

[1]As defined in this report, health outcome measures for performance partnership grants include health status, social functioning, and consumer satisfaction. For PPG purposes, risk status measures are considered to be "intermediate outcome" measures when there is a demonstrable link between the action taken to reduce a risk (e.g., vaccinations) and the desired health status outcome.

in evaluating performance in subpopulations, such as high-risk population(s). Such populations can be defined demographically, such as minorities, children, or elderly persons; by conditions, such as the lack of health insurance or homelessness; or by geographic area, such as central cities, high-risk neighborhoods, or rural communities. Specific sets of target populations can vary across states. Rather than trying to anticipate multiple submeasures that can be developed for each potential measure, the panel chose to develop broad population measures that can be tailored by each state to focus on its specific population group priorities. Clearly, validity, sample size, and other statistical issues need to be examined separately for every subpopulation.

The health outcome measures presented in this report are not meant as a mandated list. Few states are likely to have data necessary to support all of them. Furthermore, state agencies have major priorities in addition to those indicated by the outcome measures listed here (e.g., injury prevention, oral health, hearing and vision, environmental health) and are responsible for administering major programs relevant to public health (e.g., Medicaid) that are not covered by this panel's mandate. Therefore, the health outcome measures presented in this report should be considered an important subset, but not an exhaustive listing, of those that will be of interest to state agencies. Indeed, it is the panel's hope that performance measure evaluation will evolve so that new health outcome measures are continuously defined, studied, and adopted.

Similarly, the process and capacity measures presented in this report are for illustrative purposes only. Since states can pursue many reasonable strategies to improve health outcomes, a prohibitively long list of process and capacity measures would be required to cover all of their reasonable program options. The panel concluded, therefore, that the most useful approach would be to provide good, representative *examples* of relevant process and capacity measures in each program area. In order to illustrate the myriad strategies available to attain a single health outcome or risk status objective, Table 3-1 provides a list of possible program strategies and corresponding process measures aimed at reducing the incidence of smoking.

A major goal of this report is to provide an analytic framework for use by the states and DHHS in assessing the appropriateness of specific outcome, process, and capacity measures proposed for PPG agreements in the future. It is anticipated that many of the measures described in this report can, in time, be modified or replaced by others that meet the panel's selection guidelines.

Although the panel began its work with expectations that it would identify a set of core measures to support the PPG process in all the states, the panel has concluded that such a set of measures cannot be selected at this time. This conclusion is based on two findings. First, data sets to generate comparable state-level estimates exist for only a few health outcome measures; for the most part, data are not comparable across states. Second, as noted above, there are many reasonable process and capacity measures that states could adopt for PPG pur-

TABLE 3-1 Examples of Program Strategies and Related Process Measures for Reducing the Incidence of Tobacco Smoking

Program Strategy	Process Measure
Limit illegal youth purchases of smoking tobacco	Percentage of vendors who illegally sell smoking tobacco to minors Percentage of communities with ordinances and regulations restricting smoking tobacco sales Number of vending machines selling smoking tobacco in locations accessible by youth Presence or absence of state or local tobacco retailer licensing system
Increase the price of tobacco products	Amount of excise tax (cents) per pack of cigarettes
Restrict smoking tobacco advertising	Percentage of communities with ordinances or regulations restricting smoking tobacco advertising Number of billboards advertising smoking tobacco close to schools and playgrounds Number of sport or entertainment events sponsored by tobacco companies
Restrict indoor tobacco smoking	Percentage of worksites (day cares, schools, restaurants, public places) that are smoke free (or have limited smoking to separately ventilated areas)
Educate children about hazards of smoking tobacco	Proportion of elementary, junior high, and high schools with age-appropriate smoking prevention activities and comprehensive curricula
Increase access or availability of smoking cessation programs	Proportion of current tobacco smokers visiting a health care provider during the past 12 months who received advice to quit Proportion of managed care organizations (or schools or obstetric and gynecological service providers) that have active smoking prevention and cessation plans
Market effective antismoking messages to the general public	Percentage of adults who can recall seeing an antismoking message during the 12 months following a media campaign

poses, and the selection of any subset of such measures would be arbitrary. Therefore, for the future, the panel recommends that DHHS (1) assist states in standardizing both health outcome measures (especially in the areas of substance abuse and mental health) and methods for collecting data and (2) sponsor empirical outcome studies related to state agency "best practices" so that a more definitive list of recommended process and capacity measures can be developed.

The rest of this chapter presents and discusses potential outcome measures of performance and examples of process and capacity measures identified by the panel and others for each of the PPG subject areas; see Appendix C for detailed descriptions, rationale, and data sources.

CHRONIC DISEASES

Prevention of chronic disease morbidity and mortality is the primary goal of many health programs, and the outcomes of these programs must be monitored. For the most part, however, chronic disease incidence and mortality data are not useful for PPG health outcome measures because the expected time period between most prevention activities and the effect of those activities on disease incidence or mortality greatly exceeds the 3-5 years of the performance grant concept. It also exceeds the time that health departments and others are generally willing to wait to assess the effectiveness of their interventions. However, the panel recommends that states continue to measure mortality from various chronic diseases (cancers, cardiovascular disease, diabetes, etc.) through the state's vital record system. The panel also recommends that states work to develop systems to better measure the incidence and prevalence of chronic diseases. With the exception of cancers in certain geographic areas, such information is generally not now available.

Since the duration of latency of most chronic diseases prevents incidence or mortality from being a useful short-term health outcome measure, potential chronic disease measures are focused on risk reduction and screening (based on the relationship of those activities to disease reduction and more effective treatment, respectively), supplemented by process measures aimed at evaluating program activities for reducing the incidence or severity of chronic diseases. The two major strategies for this approach are reduction of the major risks leading to the development of chronic diseases and improvement of the delivery of clinical preventive services for early detection of chronic diseases.

The list of major risk reduction strategies for chronic diseases is short: prevention of tobacco use, improved nutrition, increased exercise, reduction of sun exposure, reduction of alcohol and other drug use, and, perhaps, avoidance of environmental carcinogens (e.g., radon). (Measures for the reduction of alcohol and other drug use are presented in a separate section of this report.) Prevention of tobacco use can be divided into reduction of personal tobacco use and reduction of exposure to second-hand smoke. Nutrition can be divided into two parts:

how much people eat (total calories) and what people eat (e.g., amounts of dietary fat, fruits, and vegetables).

The list of commonplace clinical preventive (or screening) services for chronic diseases that have been empirically shown to improve population outcomes or for which there is consensus regarding efficacy is also fairly short: screening for hypertension, cholesterol, breast cancer, cervical cancer, colon cancer, and osteoporosis.

In contrast to some other areas, there is a fair amount of standardization of existing measures and data collection methodologies across states in the area of chronic disease. As a consequence, the panel suggests a relatively precise set of measures for which data are widely available. For purposes of clarity, measures were defined according to the language used by the currently available survey questionnaires, as well as the populations surveyed by the commonly used methodologies. Given this construct, several possible measures, including ones for dietary fat content, sun exposure, and osteoporosis screening were not included at this time because of a current lack of data or methodology for collecting needed information.

The suggested measures do not include chronic disease treatment, such as for cardiovascular disease, chronic obstructive lung disease, cancer, etc. Screening for complications of diabetes was one exception: the panel included it because of the body of evidence showing the effectiveness of such screening, the existence of a large federal diabetes program, and the similarity in barriers and strategies for implementing these services and common general clinical preventive services.

Potential Risk Status Measures

Risk status measures represent intermediate health outcomes (see fn. 1).

Tobacco

Individual adult	Percentage of (a) persons aged 18-24 and (b) persons aged 25 and older currently smoking tobacco
Individual youth	Percentage of persons aged 14-17 (grades 9-12) currently smoking tobacco
Individual pregnant woman	Percentage of women who gave birth in the past year and reported smoking tobacco during pregnancy
Individual working adult	Percentage of employed adults whose workplace has an official policy that bans smoking

Nutrition

Content
: Percentage of persons aged 18 and older who eat five or more servings of fruits and vegetables per day[2]

Content
: Percentage of persons aged 14-17 (grades 9-12) who eat five or more servings of fruits and vegetables per day[3]

Total calories
: Percentage of persons aged 18 and older who are 20 percent or more above optimal body mass index[4]

Exercise

Individual adult
: Percentage of persons aged 18 and older who do not engage in physical activity or exercise

Individual youth
: Percentage of persons aged 14-17 (grades 9-12) who do not engage in physical activity or exercise

Screenings and Tests

Hypertension
: Percentage of persons aged 18 and older who had their blood pressure checked within past 2 years[5]

Cholesterol
: Percentage of women aged 45 and older and men aged 35 and older who had their cholesterol checked within past 5 years[6]

Breast Cancer
: Percentage of women aged 50 and older who received a mammogram within past 2 years[7]

Colon Cancer
: Percentage of adults aged 50 and older who had a fecal occult blood test within past 12 months or a flexible sigmoidoscopy within past 5 years[8]

---

[2]The numerical value in this measure is the level that is generally regarded as appropriate by the medical community; it does not represent a level that has been independently determined or endorsed by the panel.

[3]See fn. 2.

[4]See fn. 2.

[5]See fn. 2.

[6]See fn. 2.

[7]See fn. 2.

[8]See fn. 2.

Cervical Cancer	Percentage of women aged 18 and older who received a Pap smear within past 3 years[9]
Diabetes	
HbA1C	Percentage of persons with diabetes who had HbA1C checked within past 12 months[10]
Foot exam	Percentage of persons with diabetes who had a health professional examine their feet at least once within past 12 months[11]
Eye exam	Percentage of persons with diabetes who received a dilated eye exam within past 12 months[12]

Examples of Process Measures

Nutrition Program Strategy: Enable children to learn healthy dietary habits

   Process Measure: Percentage of schools with menus that meet dietary guidelines for fat content and five or more servings of fruits and vegetables daily[13]

Physical Activity Program Strategy: Increase opportunities for sedentary working adults to exercise

   Process Measure: Percentage of worksites with worksite wellness programs that include physical exercise

Smoking Program Strategy: See Table 3-1

Screening Program Strategy: Educating patients regarding need for and appropriate timing of screening tests

   Process Measure: Percentage of persons with diabetes receiving diabetes health education

---

[9]See fn. 2.
[10]See fn. 2.
[11]See fn. 2.
[12]See fn. 2.
[13]See fn. 2.

Screening Program Strategy: Improving access to screening services

Process Measure: Percentage of managed care organizations in which patients can schedule mammograms at convenient times for them

Screening Program Strategy: Implementing tracking and recall systems

Process Measure: Proportion of providers with chart-based or other real-time system for identifying women in need of mammography

Examples of Capacity Measures

Resources

Number of full-time health department employees for chronic disease prevention

Number of public service messages prepared by state agency shown annually for chronic disease prevention

Proficiencies

Number of key surveillance systems and data sets (i.e., death certificates, cancer registry data, birth certificates, Behavioral Risk Factor Surveillance System (BRFSS), Youth Risk Behavior Surveillance System (YRBSS), hospital discharge data, Medicaid and Medicare encounter information and other relevant local data sets) that are established and maintained

Percentage of local health departments receiving technical assistance and training

Percentage of labs that meet quality standards

Planning

Percentage of population served by systematic community planning process, with leadership provided by the official health agency and participation of all relevant groups (e.g., consumers, providers, advocators)

Percentage of population covered by written comprehensive chronic disease prevention plan(s) containing priorities and objectives based on needs, resources, and local demands

Community Involvement

Percentage of health care providers working under agreements established with public health departments to provide population-based prevention programming to reduce major risk factors for premature morbidity and mortality

Proportion of health department programs that operate within the framework of a community coalition or have a community advisory group

STDS, HIV, AND TUBERCULOSIS

The long-term goal for prevention efforts directed against sexually transmitted diseases (STDs) are similar to those directed against human immunodeficiency virus (HIV) infections and tuberculosis, namely, the reduction of the suffering, complications, and loss of life that these infections cause. HIV infection, tuberculosis, and many of the STDs have a natural history that resembles noninfectious chronic diseases. For some of the STDs, and certainly for HIV infection and tuberculosis, the interval between the acquisition of infection and the development of serious consequences may be years (e.g., between cervical human papilloma virus infection and cervical cancer, between HIV infection and serious immune deficiency (AIDS), and between tuberculosis infection and cavitary lung disease). Monitoring the long-term consequences of these infections is important, but their tracking does not provide a useful short-term indication of the performance of prevention efforts.

However, not all of the manifestations of these infections are delayed in onset. Acute symptomatic diseases caused by some of the STDs, many of the bacterial forms of which are completely curable by antibiotics, occur shortly after the onset of infection, and reporting these acute syndromes can provide a valid indicator of the true incidence of new infections. For tuberculosis, a small proportion of new cases develop pulmonary disease early in the course of the infection. There does not appear to be a similarly easily identifiable acute condition that occurs early in the course of HIV infection. Also, even some of the serious complications of STDs may occur relatively soon after the onset of infection (e.g., pelvic inflammatory disease and epididymitis due to gonococcal or chlamydial infection). When HIV infection (and some STDs) occur during pregnancy, the vertical transmission of the infectious agent to the fetus or newborn may also result in serious consequences relatively early in the course of the maternal infection. Indicators that measure the prevention of this vertical transmission provide potentially valid measures of prevention efforts.

For these reasons, measuring progress in this public health area is more complex than it is for other areas (e.g., immunization). Similarly, selecting useful performance measures is difficult and complex, for several reasons related to the communicable nature and the typical courses of these diseases:

1. The duration of the infectious state once the infection has occurred in an individual is often very long. (The typical duration is unique to each disease.)

2. A substantial proportion of people with new STD, HIV, or tuberculosis infections remain free of symptoms for long periods of time.

3. Even people with a newly acquired STD who do develop symptoms that prompt medical treatment will typically experience a presymptomatic interval (technically, the incubation period) during which they may be infectious to others.

4. Effective treatment is available for many of these infections, which not only benefits the individual treated by curing the infection, but also prevents the spread of the infection to others in the population.

5. Community spread of these infections appears to be maintained by a population of "core transmitters."

6. The prevention value of early diagnosis and treatment of core transmitters is substantially higher than similar efforts for the general population.

7. The predominant proportion of the spread of STDs and HIV infection in a community involves intimate sexual practices that are the object of considerable stigma in modern American society. Tuberculosis is associated with marginal and disenfranchised populations, thus bringing its own stigma. Stigma influences medical practice and reporting behaviors.

A recent Institute of Medicine (1997a) report emphasizes three major strategies for preventing STDs: reducing the risk of exposure, reducing the probability that an exposed person becomes infected, and reducing the duration of the infectious state among persons who become infected. These three general strategies apply to not only STDs, but also to HIV infection and tuberculosis, although the emphasis on each approach varies by disease. The outcome indicator best suited to measuring the results of the first two strategies seeks to measure directly, or indirectly, the incidence of disease (i.e., the rate of new infections in a defined population in a defined period of time). Prevalence monitoring (i.e., the counting of existing infections in a defined population) best measures the third approach. Indicators of incidence and of prevalence are interrelated because, all other things being equal, prevalence depends on the incidence and the duration of infection.

Potential health outcome indicators include those that attempt to measure incidence or monitor prevalence in a defined population. Indicators that attempt to measure important risk factors closely linked to disease incidence or prevalence, such as sexual behaviors, drug and alcohol use, or behaviors related to seeking medical treatment, are candidates for related outcome indicators. When these reductions can be measured in the core transmitter populations, they may be good candidates for risk status or intermediate outcome measures, as long as the data source(s) for such measures are based on sufficiently large samples to enable valid inferences to be drawn. Lastly, there are a group of indicators contingent on adequate and early treatment of cases, which can be closely linked to the prevention of further transmission, including the vertical transmission to fetuses or newborns, either before or during childbirth. Some of these indicators may prove to be useful intermediate outcome indicators.

There are no reliable direct measures of the incidence of STDs, HIV infection, and tuberculosis in the general population. Rarely are patients or health providers able to determine the exact onset of an infection. The rate of reported cases of these infections as a part of routine communicable disease surveillance is influenced not only by the true incidence of the disease, but also by the likelihood that the infected individual seeks medical care, is tested or screened, receives the correct diagnosis, and finally, is reported in the surveillance system. Consequently, state communicable disease reporting systems, particularly when associated with laboratory reporting, can be used to monitor incidence rates for some diseases, but only with a full appreciation of the potential pitfalls of these systems. In the future, some states may be able to reliably measure the incidence of reported genital herpes. The panel has selected several illustrative examples of incidence measures that may be useful to assess how a particular state is performing in its prevention efforts for STDs and HIV infection. Unfortunately, the panel is unable to suggest any incidence measure for tuberculosis since the long latency period of the disease, combined with an absence of early or intermediate symptoms, makes any incidence measure of confirmed cases inappropriate for use in performance agreements that cover 3-5 years.

Monitoring of prevalence over an extended period of time in defined populations is a very attractive potential outcome measure. In reality, trends in empirically measured prevalence may be heavily influenced by factors other than the true prevalence—such as media campaigns aimed at encouraging groups to be tested, improved laboratory screening tests, and changes in medical practice. But, very focused prevalence monitoring may provide a useful outcome indicator for the effectiveness of prevention efforts, particularly when the monitoring occurs consistently over time at sites that serve the core populations.

One additional outcome-related indicator seems advisable for prevention programs for STDs, HIV infection, and tuberculosis because they are so inextricably linked to the quality of clinical care: measurement of client satisfaction with the services being provided. Measurement of client satisfaction is particularly relevant to core transmitters. Again, special surveys of client satisfaction will have to be conducted of these populations for states interested in using this outcome measure.

Just as reduction in the prevalence of tobacco use is a valuable risk-related outcome indicator of prevention progress against lung cancer and heart disease, changes in sexual behavior, alcohol use, and condom use—particularly among core transmitters—provide potentially valuable risk-related outcome measures for STDs and HIV infection. One key difference exists, however: for tobacco use, the value of reducing smoking is quite similar for most of the population; for STDs and HIV infection, however, the general population benefit from sexual behavior risk reduction will be much greater when it occurs in the core transmitter population. Stated another way, considerable change in high-risk sexual behavior (or condom use) in a population at relatively low risk of infection might produce little demonstrable benefit in reducing incidence or prevalence in the population. Consequently, it is very important that measures of reduction of high risk sexual behavior, for example, be focused on the core groups. Similar arguments apply to reduction of injection drug use as an outcome indicator for HIV infection. A key challenge facing states that are interested in monitoring their progress in reducing the incidence of STDs and HIV infection among high-risk populations is that of small numbers: state population surveys such as BRFSS typically do not have sufficiently large samples for populations most at risk for STD and HIV transmission. In all likelihood, states that are interested in using such incidence measures will have to supplement or modify the sampling design of the BRFSS or conduct their own surveys.

Early, effective, and complete treatment of STDs and tuberculosis are essential hallmarks of preventing further spread in the community. As new therapies emerge for HIV, measurements of this outcome indicator may become important for HIV infection in the near future, as has already occurred for perinatal transmission of HIV. Intrapartum antiviral treatment, followed by treatment of the infant, is a risk status indicator of the prevention of HIV infection in newborns; similarly, standard treatment of pregnant women infected by syphilis prevents congenital syphilis.

In summary, there are three types of health outcome related measures available to states for performance agreements with DHHS in the areas of STDs, HIV infection, and tuberculosis: health status indicators (disease incidence and prevalence rates), consumer satisfaction, and risk status indicators (including completion of treatment).

Potential Health Status Outcome Measures

Incidence rates of selected STDs	Rate of reported gonococcal urethritis in men.
	Rate of reported chlamydial urethritis in men[14]
	Rate of reported cases of primary and secondary syphilis[15]
	Rate of reported cases of congenital syphilis[16]

---

[14]Can be used in states where chlamydial testing in men with urethritis is routinely performed and reported.

[15]Because of the small number of reported syphilis cases, the incidence rate will be extremely unstable.

[16]See fn. 15.

Incidence rates of HIV infection	Rate of reported newly diagnosed cases of HIV infection Rate of perinatally acquired HIV infection of infants
Prevalence rates of selected STDs	Prevalence rate of gonococcal infection in women in defined populations Prevalence rate of chlamydial infection in defined populations[17] Prevalence rate of syphilis in defined risk groups, e.g., pregnant women[18] Prevalence rate of rectal gonococcal infection in men
Prevalence rate of HIV infection	Seroprevalence of HIV infection in defined populations at high risk of the infection, e.g., pregnant women who abuse drugs

Potential Consumer Satisfaction Outcome Measure

Rates of consumer satisfaction with STD, HIV, and tuberculosis treatment programs

Potential Risk Status Measures

Risk status measures represent intermediate health outcomes (see fn. 1).

Rates of sexual activity among adolescents aged 14-17
Rates of sexual activity with multiple sex partners among people aged 18 and older
Rates of condom use during last episode of sexual intercourse among sexually active adolescents aged 14-17
Rates of condom use by persons aged 18 and older with multiple sex partners during last episode of sexual intercourse
Rates of condom use during last episode of sexual intercourse among men having sex with men
Rates of injection drug use among adolescents and adults
Completion rates of treatment for STDs, HIV infection, and tuberculosis

---

[17]See fn. 14.
[18]See fn. 15.

Examples of Process Measures

Program Strategy: Reduce barriers to receiving treatment from specific providers

Process Measure: Percentage of patients with insurance coverage for specific treatments

Process Measure: Percentage of patients reporting no transportation barriers to obtain necessary services

Process Measure: Percentage of physicians and other care providers receiving cultural competency training

Program Strategy: Improve quality of services provided

Process Measure: Percentage of cases followed up after most recent contact

Process Measure: Percentage of known intravenous drug users with access to needle exchange program

Examples of Capacity Measures

Resources

Percentage of high-risk communities with nearby testing and screening services from multiple types of health providers and public health organizations

Planning

Percentage of the state's population who reside in communities that are engaged in formal community processes for assessing and planning for HIV/STD/TB prevention and treatment services.

A primary challenge for the future is the development of accepted generalizable methodology to capture such information in high-risk target groups (e.g., injection drug users, men who have sex with men). Currently, these groups are poorly defined, disaffiliated, and difficult to reach, but there is broad consensus on the desired primary health outcome measures for these diseases (i.e., reductions of the incidence rates). The ability to accurately monitor these rates will require improved disease surveillance systems. Improvements will also have to be made in population survey methodologies used to assess risk behaviors. Greater standardization is also needed in order to improve comparability among states. Finally, there is a clear need for better integration and tracking of STD and HIV cases. Lack of integration affects treatment of individuals, identification of their contacts, and the completeness of disease surveillance and tracking. It is complicated further when each disease is treated separately. Many providers are trained to screen or treat narrowly defined classes of diseases: e.g., a respiratory specialist might treat tuberculosis, but fail to diagnose STDs or HIV infection in some patients.

MENTAL HEALTH

Many consumers, advocates, providers, and federal and state officials support the development of outcome measures for mental health in order to increase accountability and performance and to address the lack of public confidence in the effectiveness of public mental health services. The development of process measures in the public mental health field has been hampered by a lack of consensus on practice standards; although some states and private providers have developed standards, there is little agreement on them. Furthermore, there are limited research findings that establish a connection between individual process activities and mental health outcomes.

Although there is little agreement on linkages between specific process and mental health outcomes, there is some agreement on the dimensions that are important in evaluating mental health services, according to information provided by the Mental Health Statistics Improvement Program and the National Association of State Mental Health Program Directors:

1. quality assurance—process activities that are thought to produce good outcomes;
2. access to services and utilization of services;
3. consumer satisfaction with services; and
4. psychological and social outcomes.

Mental health PPG agreements should consider measures in all of these dimensions.

There are two distinct populations to be considered with respect to mental health outcomes: the consumers of mental health services and those in the general population who may or may not be consumers. Mental health providers have typically focused on outcomes for consumers, while mental health epidemiologists have focused on population outcomes. Because of limited resources, public mental health programs give priority to individuals with serious mental illnesses that require hospitalization or long-term outpatient treatment. However, population outcomes should be used when the measurement reflects an appropriate responsibility of the public mental health system, such as the number of homeless people who have a serious mental illness.

The measures presented below should be part of a future set of national mental health performance indicators; however, at this time, data to support these measures are collected only in a limited number of states and, in most cases, they are not collected in a uniform fashion. Although data for any one of the measures selected by the panel may not be available for more than a few states, any of the measures could be used as part of performance agreement for a given state as long as it reflects a priority of that state. Given the lack of nationwide data for most of these measures, the inconsistencies in how states collect data on particular measures, and the variability in use of the federal mental health block grant funds, flexibility will be required in the final PPG measures negotiated with each state. As in the other areas covered in this report, the outcome and risk status measures listed below for mental health are *not* meant to serve as a mandatory set of measures for all states over the next 3-5 years; rather, it is expected that states will select those that reflect their program priorities and can be supported by available data resources. Over time, states should endeavor to collect this information in a standard manner in order to increase its utility and comparability. Although the measures listed below are a subset of those that might be developed in the future, they would be among the least expensive to collect and would provide some of the most useful information to evaluate the adequacy of mental health services. These measures are consistent with the values associated with recovery.

Potential Health Status Outcome Measure

Percentage of persons aged 18 and older receiving mental health services who experience reduced psychological distress

Potential Social Functioning Outcome Measures

Percentage of persons aged 18 and older receiving mental health services who experience increased level of functioning

Percentage of persons aged 18 and older receiving mental health services who report increased employment (including volunteer time)

Percentage of persons aged 18 and older with serious and persistent mental illness receiving mental health services who live in integrated, independent living situations or with family members

Percentage of children aged 17 and younger with serious emotional disorders receiving mental health services who live in noncustodial living situations

Percentage of persons aged 18 and older with serious mental illness who are in prisons and jails

Percentage of children aged 17 and younger with serious emotional disorders who are in juvenile justice facilities

Percentage of homeless persons aged 18 and older who have a serious mental illness

Potential Consumer Satisfaction Outcome Measures

Percentage of adolescents aged 14-17 or family members of children and adolescents or both who are satisfied with: (a) access to services, (b) appropriateness of services, and (c) perceptions of gain in personal outcomes

Percentage of persons (aged 18 and older) or their family members or both who are satisfied with: (a) access to mental health services, (b) appropriateness of services, and (c) perceptions of gain in personal outcomes

The measures involving homelessness and living in jail or juvenile justice facilities cannot be affected, in the short run, solely by the actions taken by the state agency for mental health services. Nevertheless, the panel believes that these population-based mental health outcome measures—when combined with related process and capacity measures that are under the direct control of these agencies—can provide useful insights regarding state progress in meeting important mental health goals. Over the long run (5-10 years), state agencies responsible for mental health services should be able to demonstrate their impact on improving these outcomes.

Examples of Process and Capacity Measures

Program Strategy: Improve access to services/utilization of services

Process Measure: Percentage of adults with serious and persistent mental illness who use health services

Process Measure: Percentage of youth with serious emotional disorders who use mental health services

Process Measure: Percentage of those who use services that are voluntary

Process Measure: Percentage of people requesting services who begin receiving services within 2 weeks of the initial request

Capacity Measure: Percentage of primary care providers who receive supplemental training in mental health services

Program Strategy: Improve quality assurance

Process Measure: Percentage of service plans that include input from consumers and family members

Process Measure: Percentage of children less than 5 years old who are screened and assessed for mental health intervention

Capacity Measure: Percentage of primary care providers who use standardized screening tools for assessing the mental health status of primary care clients

The development of performance indicators for mental health should be part of a national effort to develop a standardized framework for evaluating mental health services. As that framework is developed and the needed research is completed, PPG indicators for mental health can be refined. In order for such refinement to occur, public and private administrators of mental health services will need to agree on specific mental health outcome measures and the mechanisms for capturing information on those outcomes across states. Additional research will also be needed to identify practice standards that result in the desired outcomes.

IMMUNIZATION

The biology and epidemiology of vaccine preventable diseases are well understood. Cases are, in general, easily identified, and health outcomes are well defined. A strong, causal relationship exists between immunization and disease prevention, and national standards and guidelines are well established and widely accepted. From a PPG perspective, clearly defined process (vaccination rate) and outcome (disease incidence rate) measures are the preferred means to assess vaccine preventable disease performance, and they are responsive to effective interventions within the 3-5 years proposed by DHHS. These measures provide policy-relevant information on population health and provide public health systems with the data required to assess program effectiveness and resource efficiency.

Many factors outside public health and health care delivery systems also have an impact on vaccination levels and disease incidence rates, such as immigration patterns and economic fluctuations. States also require measures to assess program effectiveness in order to facilitate adoption of effective and cost-effective interventions and to identify and terminate ineffective or inefficient programmatic initiatives. Thus, capacity and program variables also may be valuable adjuncts of immunization measures.

Although vaccination rates are risk reduction measures, the validity of their relationship to target health status outcomes is direct, proven, and universally accepted as a valid and reliable intermediate outcome measure. Indeed, given the episodic and unpredictable nature of outbreaks of vaccine-preventable diseases, a strong argument can be made that vaccination rates are a better measure of program performance than are direct measures of disease incidence. In addition to the fact that disease outbreaks are sporadic and somewhat random, the infrequency of cases is such that it may not be possible to develop statistically reliable state and metropolitan area estimates. Thus, while incident cases are relatively specific (their occurrence generally indicates a problem), sensitivity is relatively low (low vaccination rates may occur without a corresponding increase in incident cases).

Potential Health Status Outcome Measures

Reported incidence rate of representative vaccine-preventable diseases

Potential Risk Status Measures

Risk status measures represent intermediate health outcomes (see fn.1).

Age-appropriate vaccination rates for target age groups for each major vaccine group:

children aged 2 years; children entering school at approximately 5 years of age
  mumps, measles, and rubella
  diphtheria-tetanus-pertussis
  polio
  hemophilus influenza B
  hepatitis B
  varicella

adults aged 65 years and older
  diphtheria-tetanus
  hepatitis B
  influenza
  pneumococcal pneumonia

Examples of Process Measures

Program Strategy: improve access to immunization services

Process Measure: Percentage of population who do not cite financial resources as a barrier to immunization

Program Strategy: Increase parent education and awareness

Process Measure: Percentage of parents with children under 18 who believe that the benefits of immunization outweigh the risks
Process Measure: Percentage of parents with children under 18 who report receiving immunization reminders from their immunization providers

For immunization, program *capacity* is, in effect, one of the core public health functions. A state's ability to monitor vaccine compliance, facilitate vaccine access, and respond to disease outbreaks depends on both its ability to coordinate data collection with private practitioners and health delivery systems and federal data collection efforts. There are currently at least ten different sources of immunization data collected by various federal agencies. Unfortunately, many of these sources suffer from various methodological limitations that compromise their value and appropriateness for the purpose of state performance measurement (e.g., inadequate sampling frames and sample sizes that preclude reliable state-level estimates for all but the largest states and metropolitan areas; unclear data validity and reliability). For infant and childhood vaccination rate estimates, the newly developed National Immunization Survey (NIS) conducted by the National Program Immunication Office in conjunction with the National Center for Health Statistics appears to meet many of the needs of the PPG program.

Other potential sources of data include statewide registries, day care and Head Start programs, school reports, the Medicare statistical system, and for health maintenance organization's (HMOs). However, these sources are not yet developed or fully implemented and standardized across states; they require validity and reliability verification and possibly new data collection and reporting structures; and they are subject to selection bias. There are no current valid and reliable data collected on adolescent vaccination. Similarly, vaccination data from BRFSS on high-risk nonelderly adults are limited to influenza and pneumococcal pneumonia. Because most candidates for influenza and pneumonia vaccines are over 65 years old, the Medicare Statistical System can provide some estimate of vaccination, although the Medicare data on immunizations administered by hospitals and HMOs are not universally available.[19] In addition, the quality of Medicare data for residents of skilled nursing homes is not clear.

State BRFSS data on adult immunizations may not be adjusted for risk, (e.g., age and presence of respiratory conditions), limiting the value of the data for benchmarking across states. The most efficient and cost-effective way to increase the available data on vaccine incidence may be to modify and expand the NIS, taking advantage of the large sampling frame to collect data on adolescents and adults. This use may require a somewhat expanded sampling frame to ensure adequate statistical power and will require the development of additional survey modules. Finally, whenever possible, coordination of data collection effort among other performance measurement efforts is highly desirable to maximize efficiency and minimize data burden and cost.

Many of the suggestions to the panel focused on programmatic process

---

[19]The current draft of Health Employer Data and Information Set (HEDIS 3.0) requires HMOs seeking accreditation from the National Committee for Quality Assurance to report on influenza immunizations for their Medicare members and for high-risk adults under age 65.

measures. Such measures may be appropriate to include as a portion of state performance measures under limited and specific conditions: e.g., to assess progress toward development and implementation of DHHS-state agreements on programmatic initiatives, such as vaccination surveillance or administration programs for women, infants, and children; statewide registry development and implementation; insurance coverage policies; and educational programs. However, the specification of such measures must await DHHS-state agreements and should be restricted to carefully specified circumstances until relevant outcome measures are available.

SUBSTANCE ABUSE

The substance abuse measures suggested to the panel had a number of common themes and fell under several distinct categories: treatment effectiveness; treatment completion; medical screening; use during pregnancy; HIV/STDs; overall use and consequences; youth use and consequences; other prevention activities; access and special needs; and general and infrastructure issues. A list of 120 suggested measures was distilled from these categories, from which the panel identified 11 health outcome (including risk reduction) measures that best met the selection criteria presented in Chapter 2, at least for some states.[20]

Although data for any one of the measures may not be available for more than a few states, such measures could be used as part of performance agreements for any state as long as the particular measure reflects a priority of that state and the specific data sources, populations, definitions, time frames, etc., are based on the data available in that state. Given the lack of nationwide data for most of these measures, as well as the variability in how states use their federal substance abuse block grant funds, some flexibility in the final PPG measures negotiated with each state will be needed. As in the other areas discussed in this report, the panel expects that states will select from among the suggested measures listed below, to the extent that the measures can be supported by their data resources and reflect program priorities. States also should be encouraged to propose other measures that meet the panel's guidelines.

It should be noted that several of the measures listed in other sections (e.g., chronic disease; prevention of disabilities; STDs, HIV infection, and tuberculosis) may also be appropriate measures in the substance abuse area. For example, the following measures could be negotiated as part of an individual state's PPG agreement if relevant to their substance abuse efforts:

---

[20]Tobacco is of increasing concern to substance abuse agencies; specific measures involving tobacco are discussed in the separate sections on chronic diseases and disabilities.

for chronic disease:	smoking during pregnancy
for STDs, HIV infection, and tuberculosis:	injection drug use during pregnancy
for disabilities:	alcohol, tobacco, or other drug use during pregnancy

States are encouraged to coordinate the measures they select in the various areas, as well as their data collection activities to measure them.

Many of the health status and risk reduction measures listed below are not affected, in the short run, solely by the actions taken by a state agency for alcohol and drug abuse. Nevertheless, these substance abuse outcome and risk reduction measures—when combined with related process and capacity measures that are under the direct control of the agencies—can provide useful insights regarding progress in reducing problems caused by alcohol and drug abuse. Over the long run (5-10 years), state agencies responsible for alcohol and other drug abuse should be able to demonstrate their agency's impact on reducing such abuse and on the resulting problems caused by these substances.

Potential Health Status Outcome Measures

Death rate of persons aged 15-65 attributed to (a) alcohol, (b) other drug use, and (c) combined agents

Percentage of emergency room encounters for alcohol or other drug-related causes[21]

Potential Social Functioning Outcome Measures

Prevalence rate of substance abuse clients who report experiencing diminished severity of problems after completing treatment as measured by the Addiction Severity Index (ASI) or a similar measure

Ratio of substance abuse clients involved with the criminal justice system before and after completing treatment

Potential Risk Status Measures

Risk status measures represent intermediate health outcomes (see fn. 1).

---

[21]Statewide estimates are not available from the available data system that supports this measure (DAWN); however, this measure should be included among those states that may choose from if they want to focus their efforts on a defined geographical area(s) as part of their performance agreements with DHHS.

Prevalence rate of adolescents aged 14-17 engaged in heavy drinking or other drug use[22]

Prevalence rate of persons aged 18 and older engaged in heavy drinking or other drug use[23]

Percentage of women who gave birth in the past year and reported using alcohol or other drugs during pregnancy

Mean age at first use of "gateway" drugs (tobacco, marijuana, alcohol)

Percentage of adolescents aged 14-17 stating disapproval of marijuana use

Percentage of adolescents aged 14-17 who report parents or guardians who communicate non-use expectations

Percentage of drug abuse clients who engage in risk behaviors related to HIV/AIDS after completing treatment plan

Examples of Process Measures

Process Measure: Percentage of pregnant women screened for substance abuse

Process Measure: Percentage of drug abuse clients screened for STDs, HIV infection, and tuberculosis during treatment

Examples of Capacity Measures

Resources

Percentage of at-risk population(s) who have access to and receive specialized services

Planning

The presence or absence of statewide prevention and treatment needs assessment study completed within last 2 years

Percentage of providers that use uniform criteria to assess and match clients to appropriate services

There will need to be continued support for data definition and collection efforts at both the state and national level in order for states to report on the

---

[22]Although the estimated incidence rate would be a more appropriate measure of state agency performance, the most suitable data source for this measure is the YRBSS, which is a population survey and, therefore, only provides estimates of prevalence.

[23]Although the estimated incidence rate would be a more appropriate measure of state agency performance, the most suitable data source for this measure is the BRFSS, which is a population survey.

proposed substance abuse measures. In particular, support for state needs assessment studies that can support valid and reliable incidence measures of alcohol and other drug use, improved student surveys, expanded behavioral risk surveys, uniform client data sets, emergency room reporting, and client follow-up data will be critical to the ability of states to report in this important area.

Some of the measures recommended in the substance abuse area are based on self-report data, either by clients during and after treatment or by a sample of the total population. Although questions are often raised about the validity and reliability of self-report data in this area, studies that have used collateral sources to verify client self-reports have found a high degree of consistency between the clients' statements and statements from significant others (Hoffman and Harrison, 1991). One extensive review of a variety of research on the validity of substance abuse clients' self-reports (Sobell and Sobell, 1986) found that as long as clients' confidentiality was ensured and questions were objective and clear, client self-reports are sufficiently valid and reliable to be used in outcome studies.

An area of particular concern to the panel is what may happen to the ability of states to report on these measures as they move toward greater use of managed care and as previously separate funding sources are merged. As an example, many managed care firms rely heavily on consumer satisfaction surveys to measure quality of care. Such surveys are not meaningful for most substance abuse clients, most of whom dislike treatment even if their problems are reduced. The effects of major changes, such as the move to managed care and the merging of various funding streams, on the quality, cost, and effectiveness of client services will be impossible to measure if adequate attention and resources are not devoted to preserving or building data systems *before* such changes are implemented. It is important to include people at the state and local levels who are most knowledgeable about substance abuse in those decisions.

SEXUAL ASSAULT, DISABILITIES, AND EMERGENCY MEDICAL SERVICES

The panel was charged by DHHS to propose candidate performance measures in three specific areas of prevention: sexual assault, disabilities, and emergency medical services. The panel has addressed this charge but recognizes that there are many other areas of prevention of concern to public health agencies such as injury prevention. The performance measures presented here may serve as useful models for measures that could be developed for other important areas of public health.

Sexual Assault

Candidate measures suggested to the panel focused on a broad range of issues related to sexual assault, from prevention to the provision of services to those who become victims of these violent acts. A basic problem with developing meaningful indicators for sexual assault prevention programs is the difficult nature of data collection and the high degree of underreporting of assault and abuse. Another fundamental problem in measuring sexual assault is that it is currently viewed by many as a criminal justice issue rather than a public health issue. The panel identified only one measure that could be used with currently available data.

Potential Health Status Outcome Measure

Incidence rate of sexual assault reported by females

This outcome measure is very unlikely to be affected solely by actions taken by the state health agency. Nevertheless, this measure—when combined with related process and capacity measures that are under the direct control of state health agencies—can provide useful insights regarding progress in reducing the incidence of this behavior. Over the long run (5-10 years), effective programs of prevention should be able to accomplish a measurable reduction in the rate of sexual assault.

Examples of Process Measures

Process Measure: Percentage of sexual assault victims receiving acute medical and psychosocial services from specially trained personnel

Process Measure: Percentage of victims receiving postvictimization services

Examples of Capacity Measures

Resources

Percentage of at-risk population(s) who have access to and receive specialized services

Percentage of counties with rape crisis centers offering hot-line and other services

Proficiencies

Number of counties with a sexual assault surveillance system

Percentage of medical and criminal justice professionals involved with sexual assault cases who have had specialized training in these fields

Percentage of elementary and secondary schools providing educational instruction on the problem of sexual assault

Percentage of perpetrators of sexual assault who receive professional counseling designed to prevent reoccurrence

Disabilities

Performance indicators suggested to the panel reflected the focus of existing CDC programs—measures targeted toward preventing those disabilities that have their onset during childhood. The suggested indicators did not address disabilities that occur as a result of occupation or chronic illness; mental retardation resulting from congenital conditions was also not discussed. The panel believes that these are critical omissions from disability prevention and will address them during the second phase of its study.

The performance measures in this report focus on preventing initial impairment of function and preventing secondary disability due to complications from lack of or inadequate rehabilitation. Many disabilities are secondary to central nervous system illness and injury and although the panel does not offer specific measures, it believes such risk status indicators as rates of helmet use by operators of motorcycles, motorbikes, and bicycles could be useful to states in monitoring their progress toward meeting important health outcome goals. Seat belt use would also be an appropriate risk status indicator. However, data systems to support these measures are not available in most states.

Potential Health Status Outcome Measure

Percentage of newborns with neural tube defects

Potential Social Functioning Outcome Measure

Percentage of persons aged 18-65 with disabilities who are in the workforce

Potential Risk Status Measures

Risk status measures represent intermediate health outcomes (see fn. 1).

Percentage of children aged 6 or younger with blood lead greater than 10 micrograms per deciliter[24]

Percentage of women who gave birth in the past year and reported using alcohol, tobacco, or other drugs during pregnancy

The panel is aware that none of these measures is likely to be affected solely

---

[24]See fn. 2.

by actions taken by a state health agency. Nevertheless, the panel believes that these outcome measures—when combined with related process and capacity measures that are under the direct control of state health agencies—can provide useful insights regarding progress in, for example, increasing the rate of disability of persons in the workforce. The panel also believes that *over the long run* (5-10 years) state health agencies should be able to demonstrate their impact on increasing the percentage of people with disabilities who are working.

Examples of Process Measures

Program Strategy: Reduce the incidence of neural tube defects

Process Measure: Percentage of (high-risk) women screened for maternal serum alpha feto protein (MSAFP)
Process Measure: Percentage of high-risk women taking periconceptual folic acid supplementation

Program Strategy: Reduce the incidence of elevated blood lead

Process Measure: Number of counties with housing regulations designed to reduce lead hazards in low-income housing rentals
Process Measure: Percentage of parents living in homes built before 1950 who can cite lead from paint as a potential health hazard to their children

Examples of Capacity Measures

Resources

Percentage of disabled population(s) who have access to and receive specialized services

Proficiencies

Number of counties offering parents early childhood education programs focused on disabilities prevention

Planning

Number of counties actively monitoring the incidence of disabilities and the impact of disabilities

State and federal programs do not have a consistent definition of disability. This lack confounds efforts to accurately identify and measure indicators related to prevention and service delivery. The panel notes with interest the efforts by the Social Security Administration through its Medical Evaluation Study to better quantify the number of people with disabilities in this country. This study will allow the development of better indicators to measure efforts to prevent and mitigate disabilities.

Emergency Medical Services

Because the panel's charge by DHHS in this area was to focus on the emergency medical services system, indicators that relate solely to medical care in the emergency departments of hospitals were not considered unless they directly affected the quality of care in the prehospital setting or the transport and bypass decisions.[25] Among the measures suggested to the panel, the range of possible indicators covered aspects of emergency services from the initial call to treatment in specialized centers; the panel found, however, that data to support these measures were not available in most states. The panel selected measures that would be available in all jurisdictions and related to nationally accepted indicators of good emergency medical system performance. However, federal funding represents only a small portion of the funding for the emergency medical systems that exist and the cost of expanding them.

Potential Health Status Outcome Measure

Percentage of persons who suffer out-of-hospital cardiac arrest who survive

Examples of Process Measures

Process Measure: Percentage of trauma patients meeting state, or regional, triage guidelines that are transported to a trauma or burn center designated by the state or regional authority or meeting other nationally recognized criteria

Process Measure: Average time from initial call to arrival of the patient at the destination hospital

Process Measure: Percentage of emergency medical service systems with medical direction

Process Measure: Percentage of inappropriate calls to 911 or the emergency medical services system

Process Measure: Percentage of patients who receive appropriate early defibrillation

Process Measure: Percentage of the population served by poison control centers

---

[25]Indicators related to prevention of injuries were also not included as part of the charge to the panel.

Examples of Capacity Measures

Resources

Percentage of the state population with access to a trauma care system that includes:

> legal authority to designate trauma centers
> authority to establish triage procedures that allow
>   prehospital personnel to bypass nearer facilities
> trauma center identification and designation
> field categorization and triage protocols
> interhospital transfer agreements
> linkage to the rehabilitation system
> system evaluation activities

Number of counties with 911 or enhanced 911 systems
Number of counties with injury prevention programs

Proficiencies

Number of counties with 911 systems that have personnel who are able to communicate with users in their language and in a culturally competent way

Planning

Number of counties that maintain databases of prehospital care reports
Number of counties that support a statewide trauma registry

In the second phase of the panel's work, development of valid outcome measures for monitoring EMS system performance will be addressed. The panel recognizes that better systems of collecting prehospital care data with linkage to posthospital outcomes will be necessary. These measures will also need to be sensitive to the diversity of coverage areas from urban to rural, and from basic to advanced levels of care.

4

Implementing Performance-Based Agreements

In considering measurement of public health performance, it is important to make a clear distinction among four possible sources of effects: (1) specific federally financed programs; (2) other state and local public health programs; (3) programs operated by nonhealth agencies that can affect health outcomes; and (4) personal, social, economic, and other factors that are not related to any program intervention. When one or more factors may affect health outcomes, assessing their relative effects is critical to understanding the role of particular public health interventions.

Several strategies are available to try to separate the effects of programmatic and nonprogrammatic variables. For example, to improve the comparability of measures of outcomes across states or over time, one can use statistical methods to adjust a state's measures for some outcomes for inherent differences in the composition of the state's population, economy, public health infrastructure, etc., and for temporary changes in aggregate conditions (e.g., phases of the business cycle). Although such approaches have been used to structure federal-state performance-based agreements in job training programs (Heckman and Hotz, 1989), little empirical research of this type has been done in areas of public health, substance abuse, or mental health. The current level of empirical knowledge of the relationship between public health interventions and outcomes is not sufficiently well developed to allow one to judge the effectiveness of a state's efforts to realize a given heath outcome objective independent of all other factors. Making appropriate statistical adjustments for sociodemographic and other relevant factors is hampered by poorly understood relationships between individual factors and health outcomes, as well as the availability of timely and appropriate data to make such adjustments in those cases in which the relationship between particular variables and outcomes has empirically been established. Another problem with making comparisons of outcomes across states is that comparable data are often not available. Similarly, accurately comparing the progress made by different states in realizing their process and capacity objectives can be extremely difficult if states choose different process and capacity measures or set different levels of accomplishment (i.e., performance objectives). Consequently, using cross-state comparisons of "performance" as the analytic basis for determining financial rewards or penalties for participating agencies may be very problematic.

Consequently, the panel concludes that performance monitoring must make use of process and capacity measures to complement available measures of outcomes. Whenever process and capacity measures are used in performance agreements, the panel recommends that the relationships between them and desired health outcomes be explicitly related to professional standards, published clinical guidelines, or other references in the professional literature. Of course, process and capacity measures selected by a state for its performance agreements should possess the same statistical attributes as outcome measures: namely, they should be valid, reliable, and responsive. Although this "multimeasure" approach will not provide public officials or consumers with conclusive evidence of the effectiveness of particular interventions, it will allow interested parties to examine actions taken by agencies to realize their objectives and suggest whether changes in the magnitude or direction of their efforts should be considered.

Certain public health outcomes of interest to the public, program administrators, and elected officials cannot be measured in the short term because of inadequate empirical knowledge, incomplete data, or insufficient time to observe change. Yet such short-term considerations should not inhibit states and localities from implementing optimal long-run strategies for addressing public health concerns. For example, a long-term perspective is needed to measure changes in behavior, such as, smoking, for which an evaluation of the outcome would require a 20-year perspective. Moreover, short-term monitoring of performance associated with specific federally funded programs does not provide an appropriate basis for assessing the full set of responsibilities of state and local health, mental health, and substance abuse agencies. Clearly, the individual diseases and health conditions that the panel studied for this report are only a subset of those diseases and conditions that are of concern to public health agencies around the country.

Over the long term, the panel believes that it would be preferable to monitor the progress made by public health agencies in a more generic and less disease-specific approach. Until that is done, monitoring performance associated with federal funding of a particular program will be complicated considerably by the fact that funding support for programs in health agencies often comes from multiple sources. The federal mental health block grant, for example, represents only about 4 percent of state mental health agency budgets, with state general revenues, private insurance, Medicaid, and local sources making up the balance. Any general outcome indicator of mental health status is highly unlikely to provide a valid estimate of how the mental health block grant, independent of other factors, affects the overall mental well-being of a states' population.

In this regard, the illustrative capacity measures in each of the health areas do not, by themselves, reflect the full set of capacities needed by a state agency responsible for public health. Even if a state fully satisfied all of the capacity measures listed in this report, it would still need what might be called a "general readiness" capacity. For example, if a public health agency is suddenly challenged with a totally unpredictable public health threat, such as occurred when the AIDS epidemic arose or when cryptosporidiosis broke out in the Midwest, it must have the ability to respond. Under the current performance measurement system, there is no way to document such a general readiness capacity.

Process and capacity measures have certain advantages over outcome measures: the data collection for them may be less expensive, they provide useful historical information, and they more appropriately address issues of program efficiency. The panel concluded that it is not possible to formulate a list of all the process and capacity measures that could cover every possible strategy that could be adopted by a state agency to meet an important health objective in the specific areas addressed in this report. Rather, the panel decided to list examples of commonly accepted strategies that are reasonable to use. For example, there are many effective strategies for reducing the spread of vaccine-preventable diseases; as long as a state adopts some reasonable strategy for increasing the immunization rate among at-risk persons, that state should be permitted to monitor the performance of its chosen strategy. If a state agency wants to use methods not on the panel's list of commonly accepted strategies, the agency should be required to explain the connection and strength of the relationship between the process or capacity and the desired outcome.

As defined in a recent RAND report (Hill et al., 1995:9):

> [accountability is a] "process to help people who expect specific benefits from a particular activity (and whose support for the effort is essential to its continuation) to judge the degree to which the activity is working in their interests so that they might sustain it, modify it, or eliminate it.

This view is particularly appropriate for performance-based agreements between states and the federal government. As discussed in this report, the technical limitations inherent in statistical measures of performance for the near term preclude using such measures as part of a hierarchical process in which one level of government holds another under tight supervision. A more appropriate and productive approach, given the current state of data availability, is the one embraced by the federal-state approach, which allows some flexibility for each state to negotiate the specific performance measures that will most accurately reflect its particular programs and data.

A potentially important use of performance indicators is to identify possible health problems that need attention in a particular state, geographic region, or subpopulation. With an agreed-upon combination of outcome, process, and capacity measures, it becomes possible to examine the need for technical assistance to those states that appear to have a problem in realizing specific objectives, because of inadequate resources, shifting demographics, or management problems. Using performance measures to signal the need for technical assistance is consistent with the National Performance Review initiative at the federal level and with the total quality management activities that are being undertaken by public and private organizations around the country.

The data infrastructure required to support performance measures needs to be strengthened. This conclusion does not mean that the areas for improvement in data standards are unique to these programs. Indeed, public health data are often superior to those available for clinical decisions about treatment of individuals and even more so for many business and social service decisions. However, as indicated throughout this report, many of the potential health outcome measures are heavily dependent on a small number of state-federal surveys, including the Behavioral Risk Factor Surveillance System (BRFSS) and the Youth Risk Behavior Surveillance System (YRBSS). Unfortunately, these surveys do not cover all states and the methods used to collect these data vary greatly across states. Because existing resources are inadequate to support a consistent and comprehensive approach, the federal government would have to provide major increases in technical assistance and financial support for infrastructure to states if the state-federal data systems are to be able to provide the quantity and quality of data necessary to implement performance agreements.

In developing data resources that will support such agreements for public health, substance abuse, and mental health, the panel recommends that DHHS work toward the goals listed below. For each goal, the panel identifies one or more steps that can be taken by the department toward that goal.

Goal 1 Work with states to identify and develop common definitions and methods that will contribute toward standardizing measurements of health outcomes, processes, and capacity in public health, substance abuse, and mental health. Common definitions and measures are important in order to promote a common language for states, the federal government, and others to use when assessing progress toward societal goals. The panel is encouraged that the Substance Abuse and Mental Health Services Administration is planning a major effort for state data infrastructure development.

Suggested Steps

Pursue strategies to improve collection and integration of public health, substance abuse, and mental health services data, particularly from capitated managed care providers.

Support research to examine the relationship between interventions (process) and specific health outcomes.

Goal 2   Encourage consolidation of data resources in ways that can efficiently support multiple programs (e.g., public health, substance abuse and mental health) and a broad range of purposes (e.g., performance monitoring, evaluation, and program operations).

Suggested Step

Encourage states and federal agencies to consolidate data resources as a means of increasing the efficiency of existing information systems and surveys.

Goal 3   Identify and respond to states' priorities for data related to public health, substance abuse, and mental health policy and practice.

Suggested Steps

Convene state program directors on a regular basis to identify data needs and discuss progress in developing appropriate information systems and data surveys.

Incorporate consideration of state data needs in the development and improvement of federal data resources.

Goal 4   Identify and promote the data collection and analytic capabilities of states with regard to public health, substance abuse, and mental health.

Suggested Steps

Identify efforts at the state level that may serve as models for other states (and national) data resource development, such as confidentiality agreements that allow different state health agencies to share client information and still protect confidentiality so that these systems can be used for statistical purposes.

Establish a grant program that will help create model state data systems.

Provide additional resources to states to promote analytic and data gathering capabilities, such as helping states develop surveys of high quality and integrate them with administrative data, so that national statistics can be built on them, and developing BRFSS and YRBSS enhancements and analysis training.

Most important, the panel recommends that using performance measures to accurately assess the effectiveness of public health, substance abuse, and mental health programs be viewed as an on-going, long-term public administration activity, with a strong federal commitment to providing technical assistance and infrastructure support to its partners at the state and local level. Although much useful information can be gathered over the next several years on health outcomes, processes, and capacities, the full utilization of performance measures to improve programs must await the development of more and better empirical information on the effect of interventions on outcomes, as well as more complete, uniform, and timely data on those outcomes. Longer term research and the development of the information systems needed to support more adequate performance measures in these areas will be the subject of the panel's second report.

References

Heckman, James, and V.J. Hotz
 1989 Choosing among alternative nonexperimental methods for estimating the impact of social programs: The case of manpower training. *Journal of the American Statistical Association* 84(December):862-880.
Hill, Paul T., James Harvey, and Amy Praskac
 1995 Dimensions of the box: Defining accountability and performance standards. Pp. 9-16 in *Pandora's Box: Accountability and Performance Standards in Vocational Education*. Santa Monica, CA: RAND.
Hoffman, N.G., and P.A. Harrison
 1991 The Chemical Abuse Treatment Outcome Registry (CATOR): Treatment outcome for private programs. Pp. 115-133 in J. Spicer, *Does Your Program Measure Up? An Addiction Professional's Guide for Evaluating Treatment Effectiveness*. Center City, MN: Hazeldon.
Institute of Medicine
 1988 *The Future of Public Health*. Committee for the Study of the Future of Public Health, Division of Health Care Services. Washington, DC: National Academy Press.
 1997a *The Hidden Epidemic: Confronting Sexually Transmitted Diseases*. Committee on Prevention and Control of Sexually Transmitted Diseases, Division of Health Promotion and Disease Prevention. Washington, DC: National Academy Press.
 1997b *Improving Health in the Community: A Role for Performance Monitoring*. Committee on Using Performance Monitoring to Improve Community Health, Division of Health Promotion and Disease Prevention. Washington, DC: National Academy Press.
 1997c *Managing Managed Care: Quality Improvement in Behavioral Health*. Committee on Quality Assurance and Accreditation Guidelines for Managed Behavioral Health Care, Division of Neuroscience and Behavioral Health, Division of Health Care Services. Washington, DC: National Academy Press.

Lewin-VHI, Inc.
  1997   *Strategies for Obtaining Public Health Infrastructure Data at Federal, State, and Local Levels.* Report to the Public Health Service. Washington, DC: U.S. Department of Health and Human Services.
National Center for Health Statistics
  1996   *Healthy People 2000 Review, 1995-1996.* Public Health Service. Washington, DC: U.S. Department of Health and Human Services.
Sobell, L.C., and M.B. Sobell
  1986   Can we do without alcohol abusers' self-reports? *The Behavior Therapist* 9:141-146.

Appendices

APPENDIX
A

Performance Measures: Source Materials

Association of State and Territorial Health Officials (ASTHO). Principles for Selecting Health Outcomes Objectives. Washington, DC. August 1995.

ASTHO suggests specific criteria to be used when choosing health outcomes objectives, including comparability, reliability, specificity, accessibility, and relevancy.

Barnow, B.S. The effects of performance standards on state and local programs. In *Evaluating Welfare and Training Programs*, C.F. Manski and I. Garfinkel, eds. Cambridge, MA: Harvard University Press. 1992.

The author discusses the issues that should be considered in developing performance standards for the Job Opportunities and Basic Skills (JOBS) program. He defines the concept of performance management as it relates to employment and training programs and discusses how a performance measurement system can help channel behavior in the direction desired by the federal government. The author reviews the Job Training Partnership Act (JTPA) and applies the lessons learned under that program to the JOBS program.

Barrett, T.J., B. Berger, and L. Bradley. Performance contracting: The Colorado model revisited. *Administration and Policy in Mental Health*, 20(2). 1992.

This article describes the performance contracting model that was developed in 1986-1987 by the Colorado Division of Mental Health (DMH) and the Colorado Association of Community Mental Health Centers and Clinics (CACMHCC). Several performance contracting issues were left unresolved, including the identification of performance indicators that focus on the quality of services provided and outcome measures, rather than process measures.

Friedlander, D. *Sub-Group Impacts and Performance Indicators for Selected Welfare Employment Programs*. New York: Manpower Demonstration and Research Corporation. 1988.

The purpose of this study of five mandatory welfare employment programs was to determine the programs' effects on employment and welfare status and to explore the validity of certain performance measures. The study found that unadjusted outcome measures (in this case, simple job-entry and case closure) are not valid indicators of performance as they tend to substantially overstate the true effects and that overstatement is not uniform across subgroups. Differences in program performance were determined more by characteristics of enrollees, local AFDC requirements, and local employment conditions than by the program.

Hansen, J. S., ed. *Preparing for the Workplace*. Committee on Postsecondary Education and Training for the Workplace, Commission on Behavioral and Social Sciences and Education, National Research Council. Washington, DC: National Academy Press. 1994.

One of the programs examined by the Committee on Postsecondary Education and Training was the Job Training Partnership Act (JTPA), a program that had a well-developed set of performance measures and goals specified in its statute. The experience of the JTPA performance measures was mixed: although they increased program credibility, they also fostered "creaming" and encouraged short-term approaches. The committee found no evidence that programs with performance standards had greater effect than those without them. The committee concluded that outcome standards are not always preferable to process measures, especially when process measures focus on "best practices."

Hatry, H., et al., *Monitoring the Outcomes of Economic Development Programs: A Manual*. Washington, DC: The Urban Institute Press. 1989.

The Urban Institute and the states of Maryland and Minnesota undertook the task of designing a performance monitoring system for selected major economic development programs. The system was designed to provide feedback on service outcomes and service quality. Some of the other system criteria were frequent and timely performance information; a focus on outcomes accruing to clients; the need for nontraditional data sources; the inclusion of both intermediate and end outcomes; an assessment of successful impacts caused by the state program; a means to compare performance over time and to previous years; and a design that minimizes the costs of data collection and management procedures. Among the limitations of the system is that performance information does not really explain why outcomes are the way they are; the best it can do is suggest reasons.

Hatry, H. State and local government productivity and performance measurement. In *State and Local Government Administration*, J. Rabin and D. Dodd, eds. New York: Marcel Dekker. 1985.

The author discusses how performance monitoring is used, including resource allocation, program planning, and contract monitoring. The author outlines several types of performance measures, including effectiveness and quality measures that assess the degree to which stated objectives are achieved and any negative consequences resulting from the service; efficiency measures, including input/output measures, work standards, and productivity indices. A major issue in performance measurement is how to assess whether what is being measured is good or bad. The author offers seven benchmarks that might be of use in making a determination: (1) existing standards, (2) previous performance, (3) the performance of similar units, (4) outcomes for different client groups, (5) performance in other jurisdictions, (6) performance of the private sector, and (7) preset targets.

Hill, P.T., J. Harvey, and A. Praskac. *Pandora's Box: Accountability and Performance Standards in Vocational Education*. National Center for Research in Vocational Education, University of California, Berkeley. Santa Monica, CA: The RAND Corporation. 1993.

In developing statewide performance standards and measures for vocational education programs, the authors state that all performance measures should be developed around at least three outcomes: learning, student success in the labor markets, and community-wide support for vocational programs. The authors argue that any accountability system must emphasize meeting local needs because only local actors can judge whether the program is operating successfully. Several impediments to effective state-local cooperation are noted, including the lack of resources and personnel to support an effective performance measurement development effort.

Hoachlander, E.G. Systems of Performance Standards and Accountability for Vocational Education: Guidelines for Development. National Center for Research in Vocational Education, University of California, Berkeley. 1991.

This monograph defines performance measures, offers guidelines as to what type of measures should be developed, what constitutes a good measure, the types of statistical controls needed, and how best to proceed to develop a system of measures.

Illinois Department of Public Health. Illinois Project for Local Assessment of Needs. Springfield. December 1993.

This paper describes a new approach to the planning and delivery of public health services in Illinois. Practice standards and performance indicators are used to measure the core functions of public health. Local health departments are required to perform needs assessments every 5 years and develop a community health plan that addresses three priority areas. Block grant funds are used to support the planning activities that will result in capacity and needs assessments. Training and technical assistance are provided by state health department staff and by a team from the Southern Illinois University at Carbondale.

Kamis-Gould, E. The New Jersey Performance Management System: A state system and uses of simple measures. *Evaluation and Program Planning*, 10:249-255. 1987.

The New Jersey Performance Management System (PMS) was developed to ascertain whether the mental health agency performance was congruent with the state mandate and if intended results were produced. Four areas of performance were identified as critical: appropriateness, adequacy, efficiency, and effectiveness. These four dimensions were repeatedly subdivided, yielding operationally defined performance indicators available from routine reports. A task force was charged with the development of the indicators along with a dictionary of terms used in the PMS, statistical and accounting guidelines to assure uniform derivation of the indicators, and statistical decisions that define high and low performance.

Larson, M.J., J.C. Buckley, and E.A. Elliott. Data Collection on Key Indicators for Policy, Alcohol, Illicit Drugs and Tobacco. Institute for Health Policy, Brandeis University. February 1995.

This paper presents detailed profiles of 34 data collection activities that can be used to monitor the nation's progress in reducing the effects linked with drugs, alcohol and tobacco. Each profile contains information on the purpose of the collection, the sponsoring agency, the type of information gathered, and the survey sample design.

Lewin-VHI, Inc. Key Monitoring Indicators of the Nation's Health and Health Care and their Support by NCHS Data Systems. Prepared for the Office of

Analysis, Epidemiology and Health Promotion, National Center for Health Statistics, Centers for Disease Control and Prevention. Fairfax, VA. April 1995.

This report describes an evaluation of the adequacy and appropriateness of information collected by NCHS to support key indicators to monitor changes in the nation's health care system. A conceptual framework for classifying and evaluating indicators is outlined, and an ideal set of indicators is identified, as is a set that can be readily obtained. The report concludes with recommendations for next steps toward the implementation of a key indicator monitoring system.

Minnesota Planning. Minnesota Milestones: 1993 Progress Report. St. Paul, MN. May 1994.

In this report Minnesota rates its progress toward measurable goals set forth in 1992. Data are compared between 1990 and 1992, and targets to be accomplished by 1995 are presented. Each goal is graded with plus or minus sign to indicate the direction of progress. Goals are broad, cover a variety of areas— such as education, health, economic growth and the environment—and represent Minnesotans' hopes for the future of their state. Attached to each goal is a set of measurable indicators. The report also describes advances made in the collection of results-oriented data.

National Association of County Health Officials. APEX*PH*: Assessment Protocol for Excellence in Public Health. Washington, DC. March 1991.

APEX*PH* is a voluntary process for community self-assessment, improvement planning, and internal evaluation by local health departments. Its purpose is to enhance organizational capacity and strengthen a department's leadership in the community so that it can better achieve goals that are relevant to that community. This workbook provides guidance in assessing and improving organizational capacity and for working with the local community to make improvements to its health status.

National Center for Health Statistics. *Healthy People 2000 Review, 1994.* Washington, DC: U.S. Department of Health and Human Services. 1995.

Healthy People 2000 is a nationwide prevention and health promotion initiative to track and improve the nation's health through the 1990s. It is a framework to reduce preventable death and disability, enhance quality of life, and reduce disparities in health status among different population groups. Objectives are organized in 22 priority areas, each with its own set of objectives. This 1994 review gives a summary of the objectives and of the progress made in meeting them.

National Center for Health Statistics. *Statistical Notes, Number 10.* Washington, DC: U.S. Department of Health and Human Services. September 1995.

One major goal of *Healthy People 2000* is to reduce health disparities among Americans, including disparities between race and ethic groups. This newsletter, based on recommendations from the Committee 22.1, presents updates for previously published trends for the Health Status Indicators for the total population and presents comparisons by race and Hispanic origin using current national data.

National Center for Health Statistics. *Statistics and Surveillance, Number 6.* Washington, DC: U.S. Department of Health and Human Services. January 1995.

This newsletter discusses the development and recommendations of the Committee 22.1, a group of health professionals, who were convened by the Centers for Disease Control and Prevention to identify a consensus set of indicators that would meet the requirements of the *Healthy People 2000* objective that calls for the development and implementation of a set of Health Status Indicators for federal, state, and local use.

North Carolina Office of State Planning. Performance measures in the performance/program budget. *Office of State Planning Newsletter* 2(1). March 1995.

This paper describes a key element of the North Carolina budget: the agency outcome measure, which is a results-oriented, numeric indicator of agency performance. Outcome measures are meaningful in the context of what an agency expects to accomplish and how it expects to reach its goals and are an integral part of an agency's strategic planning process and program management. Teams of staff members in each department developed a single measure for each outcome in the budget. Office of State Planning staff worked with the teams to ensure that the measures were statistically reliable and valid.

Oregon Commission on Children and Families. Communities Investing in the Future, 1994 Comprehensive Planning Guide. Portland, OR. 1994.

This document presents a step-by-step guideline designed to assist Oregon counties as they develop a mandated comprehensive plan for the well-being of all the children in that county. Steps include "community mapping" (needs assessment), selection of core benchmarks, identification of short- and long-term goals, and the development of a macro budget to implement the plan.

Oregon Option. The Oregon Option: A Proposed Model for Results-Driven Intergovernmental Service Delivery. Portland, OR. July 1994.

This paper describes a proposed demonstration project that would be a partnership between Oregon and the federal government to redesign public service delivery based on measurable outcomes. Both the state and federal government will identify results to be achieved and the state will contract to achieve them. Both partners will agree to merge funding streams, renegotiate funding levels, eliminate costly restrictions and provide multi-year funding. The demonstration project will focus initially on the Oregon benchmarks that address economic and social concerns.

Oregon Progress Board. Oregon Benchmarks: Standards for Measuring Statewide Progress and Institutional Performance. Report to the 1995 Legislature. Portland, OR. December 1994.

This report describes the Oregon benchmarks, statutorily mandated, measurable indicators that the state uses to chart its progress towards broad strategic goals. Those goals are for its citizens to be educated, functioning people, working in well-paid jobs, and living in thriving communities. The benchmark system allows Oregon to have and pursue long-range goals while keeping tabs on the immediate problems. This is achieved by a focus on measurable outcomes as indicators of achievement rather than a focus on programs and expenditures.

Special Study Panel on Educational Indicators. *Education Counts: An Indicator System to Monitor the Nation's Health.* Washington, DC: U.S. Department of Education. 1991.

The panel was asked to define specific indicators to assess the nation's educational performance. It developed indicators around six issue areas: learner outcomes, quality of educational institutions, readiness for school, education and economic productivity, equity, and societal support for living. Several obstacles were identified as barriers to indicator development: (1) a lack of consensus on a conceptual model of an optimally functioning system; (2) problems with validity and reliability, e.g., large gaps in data sources; (3) the need to ensure fair comparisons among schools and students; (4) time and resource burdens imposed by the implementation of an indicator system; and (5) local pressures to produce desired statistical outcomes.

Stantitis, T. Review and Analysis of Alcohol and Drug Abuse Performance Agreements in California, Michigan, and Oregon. National Association of State Alcohol and Drug Abuse Directors (NASADAD). Washington, DC. 1996.

This project reviews the performance contracts used by California, Michigan, and Oregon to provide services to counties and community-based treatment programs. Reviewers found that each state handles their performance agreements differently in the areas of contractor selection, data management, fiscal processes and methods of incentives or negative repercussions. The report suggested lessons that could be learned and recommended specific courses of action.

Substance Abuse and Mental Health Services Administration. *Developing State Outcomes Monitoring Systems for Alcohol and Other Drug Abuse Treatment.* Treatment Improvement Protocol Series 14, DHHS Publication No. (SMA) 95-3031. Washington, DC: U.S. Department of Health and Human Services. 1995.

Outcomes-based monitoring systems are broad-based efforts that link data from a variety of alcohol and drug programs. This treatment improvement protocol is designed to help state agencies to develop, implement, and manage their systems to improve treatment outcomes and increase accountability for substance abuse treatment funding. In addition to outlining the methods and technical concerns involved in developing a monitoring system, the volume offers a discussion of the political and ethical considerations.

Substance Abuse and Mental Health Services Administration. Outcomes Monitoring Planning Group Meeting: Report on the Second Working Meeting of the Center for Substance Abuse Treatment. Washington, DC. November 16, 1995.

This report of a meeting of state directors and their research and data experts continues the development of outcomes monitoring measures appropriate for state substance abuse agencies. The group reached consensus on a set of state-specific objectives in the areas of accessibility to services, process, outcomes, and societal impact. Recommendations were made on state and national data sources and on the steps needed to set up a feasibility study.

U.S. General Accounting Office. *Program Performance Measures: Federal Agency Collection and Use of Performance Data.* Washington, DC: U.S. General Accounting Office, GAO/GGD-92-65. 1992.

This survey of 103 federal agencies covered the current state of performance measures, i.e., to what extent measures have been developed and how are they used. Three-quarters of the agencies surveyed reported that they collected a variety of data to assess performance. Types of measures collected included inputs, workload, outputs, outcomes, and efficiency measures.

U.S. Department of Health and Human Services. Guiding Principles for Selecting Performance Partnership Objectives. Draft technical document excerpted from Examples of Prototype Performance Partnership Objectives. Washington, DC. May 1995.

This document offers ten guidelines for selecting partnership objectives and urges that they draw on *Healthy People 2000* whenever appropriate. Guidelines are designed to make the objectives understandable and measurable.

U.S. Office of Management and Budget. *Performance Partnerships: Guiding Principles*. Washington, DC: U.S. Office of Management and Budget. 1994.

OMB suggests that performance measures be a mix of outcome and output measures and be mutually developed by those involved along with the federal government. Measures need to specify performance information, data sources, acceptable levels of precision and accuracy, domain of measurement, frequency of data collection, and period of time covered. Measures should be refined over time.

Washington State Department of Health. Public Health Improvement Plan, A Progress Report. Olympia, WA. March 1994.

This report describes the Washington Public Health Improvement Plan, a blueprint to improve the health status of the state through prevention and capacity development for public health services. It is based on specific objectives across a range of public health activities and lists outcome standards for each area. The report also details what capacity is needed to meet these standards as well as other interventions needed to improve the health status of Washington's citizens.

B

Overview of Federal Data Sources
for PPG Measures

The table in this appendix presents information about almost 50 federal databases that are potential data sources for performance monitoring, from 11 agencies in 5 departments.

TABLE B-1 Potential Data Sources for Performance Monitoring

Federal Database	Department	Agency	Data Type
AIDS Surveillance System	DHHS	CDC	Report
Annual Census of Patient Characteristics: State and County Mental Health Inpatient Services	DHHS	SAMHSA	Census
Annual Survey of Occupational Injuries and Illnesses	DOL	BLS	Survey
Area Resource File (ARF)	DHHS	HRSA	Record
Behavioral Risk Factors Surveillance System (BRFSS)	DHHS	CDC	Survey
Consumer Expenditure Survey	DOL	BLS	Survey
Current Population Survey, Tobacco Use Supplement	DOC	BOC	Survey
Current Population Surveys (CPS)	DOC	BOC	Survey
Decennial Census of the U.S. Population	DOC	BOC	Census
Drug Abuse Warning Network (DAWN)	DHHS	SAMHSA	Report
Drug Use Forecasting Program (DUF)	DOJ	NIJ	Survey
Fatal Accident Reporting System (FARS)	DOT	NHTSA	Report
Healthcare Cost and Utilization Project (HCUP): Nationwide Inpatient Sample (NIS)	DHHS	AHCPR	Record
Healthcare Cost and Utilization Project (HCUP): State Inpatient Database (SID)	DHHS	AHCPR	Record
Inventory of Mental Health Organizations and General Hospital Mental Health Services	DHHS	SAMHSA	Survey
Inventory of Mental Health Services in the Criminal Juvenile Justice Systems	DHHS	SAMHSA	Survey
Linked Files of Live Birth and Infant Death Records	DHHS	CDC	Record
Medicaid Data System (MDS)	DHHS	HCFA	Record
Medical Expenditure Panel Survey (MEPS)	DHHS	AHCPR	Survey
Medicare Statistical Data System	DHHS	HCFA	Record
Monitoring the Future Survey	DHHS	NIH	Survey

Data Collection Frequency	Geographic Coverage				Similar State System[b]
	Nat'l	All States	Some States	Other[a]	
Continuous	x	x		x	x
Annual			x		x
Annual	x	x			
Continuous	x	x		x	x
Annual+		x			x
Annual	x		x		
Every 2 years	x	x			
Monthly	x		x		
Decennial	x	x		x	
Continuous				x	
Quarterly				x	
Continuous	x	x		x	x
Ongoing	x				
Ongoing			x		x
Every 2 years	x	x			x
Periodic		x			x
Annual	x	x		x	x
Continuous	x	x			x
Continuous	x		x		
Continuous	x	x			x
Annual	x			x	

continued on next page

TABLE B-1   Continued

Federal Database	Department	Agency	Data Type
National Ambulatory Medical Care Survey (NAMCS)	DHHS	CDC	Survey
National Facility Register (NFR)	DHHS	SAMHSA	Survey
National Health Interview Survey (NHIS)	DHHS	CDC	Survey
National Home and Hospice Care Survey	DHHS	CDC	Survey
National Hospital Ambulatory Medical Care Survey	DHHS	CDC	Survey
National Hospital Discharge Survey	DHHS	CDC	Record
National Household Survey on on Drug Abuse	DHHS	SAMHSA	Survey
National Immunization Survey (NIS)	DHHS	CDC	Survey
National Judicial Reporting System	DOL	BLS	Survey
National Mortality Followback Survey	DHHS	CDC	Survey
National Notifiable Diseases Surveillance System (NNDSS)	DHHS	CDC	Report
National Nursing Home Survey (NNHS)	DHHS	CDC	Survey
National Program of Cancer Registries	DHHS	CDC	Record
National Survey of Ambulatory Surgery	DHHS	CDC	Survey
National Survey of Childbearing Women	DHHS	CDC	Survey
National Traumatic Occupational Fatalities Surveillance System	DHHS	CDC	Record
National Vital Statistics System	DHHS	CDC	Record
Pregnancy Risk Assessment Monitoring System (PRAMS)	DHHS	CDC	Survey
Sample Surveys of Clients/Patients in Mental Health Organizations and General Hospital Psychiatry Services	DHHS	SAMHSA	Survey
State Profile System	DHHS	SAMHSA	Survey
State Trauma Registries	DHHS	HRSA	Record
Surveillance, Epidemiology, and End Results Program (SEER)	DHHS	NIH	Record
Survey of Income and Program Participation (SIPP)	DOC	BOC	Survey

Data Collection Frequency	Geographic Coverage				Similar State System[b]
	Nat'l	All States	Some States	Other[a]	
Annual	x			x	x
Annual	x	x			
Annual	x		x		x
Annual	x			x	x
Annual	x				x
Annual	x				x
Periodic	x				
Continuous	x	x			x
Every 2 years	x				
Periodic	x				
Continuous	x	x			x
Periodic	x				x
Continuous			x		x
Ongoing	x				x
Ongoing (on hold)			x		
Continuous	x	x			x
Continuous	x	x		x	x
Monthly			x	x	x
Periodic	x		x		x
Annual		x			x
Annual	x	x			x
Continuous				x	x
Periodic	x				

continued on next page

TABLE B-1 Continued

Federal Database	Department	Agency	Data Type
Treatment Episode Data Set (TEDS) (formerly, Client Data Systems)	DHHS	SAMHSA	Report
Uniform Crime Reporting (UCR) Data	DOJ	FBI	Census
Uniform Facility Data Set (UFDS)	DHHS	SAMHSA	Survey
Youth Risk Behavior Surveillance System (YRBSS)	DHHS	CDC	Survey

[a]Available for region, metropolitan area, or other nonstate geographic area.

[b]Data originated from state-initiated data collection effort or state collects data similar to federal effort.

ABBREVIATIONS:

Federal Departments

DHHS	Department of Health and Human Services
DOC	Department of Commerce
DOJ	Department of Justice
DOL	Department of Labor
DOT	Department of Transportation

Federal Agencies

AHCPR	Agency for Health Care Policy and Research
BLS	Bureau of Labor Statistics
BOC	Bureau of the Census
CDC	Centers for Disease Control and Prevention
FBI	Federal Bureau of Investigation
HCFA	Health Care Financing Administration
HRSA	Health Resources and Services Administration
NHTSA	National Highway Traffic Safety Administration
NIH	National Institutes of Health
NIJ	National Institute of Justice
SAMHSA	Substance Abuse and Mental Health Services Administration

Data Collection Frequency	Geographic Coverage				Similar State System[b]
	Nat'l	All States	Some States	Other[a]	
Monthly-quarterly			x		x
Monthly	x	x		x	x
Annual			x		x
Every 2 years	x		x		x

C
Potential Health Outcome and Risk Status Measures

The health outcome and risk status measures in this appendix are presented to illustrate the types of measures that might be included in performance partnership grants (PPG) between state agencies and the U.S. Department of Health and Human Services (DHHS). These measures were selected from among the many proposed to the panel by participants at four regional meetings sponsored by DHHS, as well as by professional health associations and private agencies and individuals. The panel chose the measures—listed in the first section of this appendix and detailed in the second section—using the guidelines described in Chapter 1 of this report: a measure should be specific and results oriented; it should be meaningful and understandable; data should be adequate to support the measure; and the measure should be as valid, reliable, and responsive as possible.

These health outcome and risk status measures are not meant to represent a mandated list. Few states are likely to have all of the data necessary to support all of these measures. In addition, state agencies may well have major priorities in addition to those represented by the categories of outcome measures listed here (e.g., injury prevention, oral health, hearing and vision, environmental health, etc.) and are responsible for administering major programs relevant to public health that are not covered by this report (e.g., Medicaid). In addition, the panel did not attempt to identify all of the measures that might be relevant for specific important subpopulations (i.e., groups defined by demographic or risk categories). Consequently, the health outcome and risk status measures described below should be considered an important subset, but not an exhaustive listing, of those that will be of interest to state agencies.

A major goal of this report is to provide an analytic framework for use by the states and DHHS in assessing the appropriateness of specific outcome, process, and capacity measures proposed for PPG agreements in the future. The panel hopes that the field of performance measure evaluation will evolve, as new health outcome measures are defined, studied, and become available. It is anticipated that many of the measures described in this report can, in time, be modified or replaced by others that meet the selection guidelines listed above.

POTENTIAL MEASURES: OVERVIEW

Chronic Disease

Tobacco

* Percentage of (a) persons aged 18-24 and (b) persons aged 25 and older currently smoking tobacco
* Percentage of persons aged 14-17 (grades 9-12) currently smoking tobacco
* Percentage of women who gave birth in the past year and reported smoking tobacco during pregnancy
* Percentage of employed adults whose workplace has an official policy that bans smoking

Nutrition

* Percentage of persons aged 18 and older who eat five or more servings of fruits and vegetables per day[1]
* Percentage of persons aged 14-17 (grades 9-12) who eat five or more servings of fruits and vegetables per day[2]
* Percentage of persons aged 18 and older who are 20 percent or more above optimal body mass index[3]

Exercise

* Percentage of persons aged 18 and older who do not engage in physical activity or exercise
* Percentage of persons aged 14-17 (grades 9-12) who do not engage in physical activity or exercise

---

[1]The numerical value in this measure is the level that is generally regarded as appropriate by the medical community; it does not represent a level that has been independently determined or endorsed by the panel.

[2]See fn. 1.

[3]See fn. 1.

Screenings and Tests

• Percentage of persons aged 18 and older who had their blood pressure checked within past 2 years[4]

• Percentage of women aged 45 and older and men aged 35 and older who had their cholesterol checked within past 5 years[5]

• Percentage of women aged 50 and older who received a mammogram within past 2 years[6]

• Percentage of adults aged 50 and older who had a fecal occult blood test within past 12 months or a flexible sigmoidoscopy within past 5 years[7]

• Percentage of women aged 18 and older who received a Pap smear within past 3 years[8]

• Percentage of persons with diabetes who had HbA1C checked within past 12 months[9]

• Percentage of persons with diabetes who had a health professional examine their feet at least once within past 12 months[10]

• Percentage of persons with diabetes who received a dilated eye exam within past 12 months[11]

STDs, HIV Infection, and Tuberculosis

• Incidence rates of selected STDs

• Incidence rates of HIV infection

• Prevalence rates of selected STDs

• Prevalence rates of HIV infection

• Consumer satisfaction with STD, HIV, and tuberculosis treatment programs

• Rates of sexual activity among adolescents aged 14-17

• Rates of sexual activity with multiple sex partners among people aged 18 and older

• Rates of condom use during last episode of sexual intercourse among sexually active adolescents aged 14-17

• Rates of condom use by persons aged 18 and older with multiple sex partners during last episode of sexual intercourse

---

[4]See fn. 1.

[5]See fn. 1.

[6]Cancer incidence by diagnosed stage may be a better alternative in cancer registry areas; see fn. 1.

[7]See fns 1 and 6.

[8]See fns. 1 and 6.

[9]See fn. 1.

[10]See fn. 1.

[11]See fn. 1.

- Rates of condom use during last episode of sexual intercourse among men having sex with men
- Rates of injection drug use among adolescents and adults
- Completion rates of treatment for STDs, HIV infection, and tuberculosis

Mental Health

- Percentage of persons aged 18 and older receiving mental health services who experience reduced psychological distress
- Percentage of persons aged 18 and older receiving mental health services who experience increased level of functioning
- Percentage of persons aged 18 and older receiving mental health services who report increased employment (including volunteer time)
- Percentage of persons aged 18 and older with serious and persistent mental illness receiving mental health services who live in integrated, independent living situations or with family members
- Percentage of children aged 17 and younger with serious emotional disorders receiving mental health services who live in noncustodial living situations
- Percentage of persons aged 18 and older with serious mental illness who are in prisons and jails
- Percentage of children aged 17 and younger with serious emotional disorders who are in juvenile justice facilities
- Percentage of homeless persons aged 18 and older who have a serious mental illness
- Percentage of adolescents aged 14-17 or family members of children and adolescents or both who are satisfied with: (a) access to services, (b) appropriateness of services, and (c) perceptions of gain in personal outcomes
- Percentage of persons (aged 18 and older) or their family members or both who are satisfied with: (a) access to mental health services, (b) appropriateness of services, and (c) perceptions of gain in personal outcomes

Immunization

- Reported incidence rate of representative vaccine-preventable diseases
- Age-appropriate vaccination rates for target age groups (children aged 2 years; children entering school at approximately 5 years of age; and adults aged 65 and older) for each major vaccine group

Substance Abuse

- Death rate of persons aged 15-65 attributed to (a) alcohol, (b) other drug use, and (c) combined agents
- Percentage of emergency room encounters for alcohol or other drug-related causes

- Prevalence rate of substance abuse clients who report experiencing diminished severity of problems after completing treatment as measured by the Addiction Severity Index (ASI) or a similar measure[12]
- Ratio of substance abuse clients involved with the criminal justice system before and after completing treatment
- Prevalence rate of adolescents aged 14-17 engaged in heavy drinking or other drug use[13]
- Prevalence rate of persons aged 18 and older engaged in heavy drinking or other drug use[14]
- Percentage of women who gave birth in the past year and reported using alcohol or other drugs during pregnancy
- Mean age at first use of "gateway" drugs (tobacco, marijuana, alcohol)
- Percentage of adolescents aged 14-17 stating disapproval of marijuana use
- Percentage of adolescents aged 14-17 who report parents or guardians who communicate non-use expectations
- Percentage of drug abuse clients who engage in risk behaviors related to HIV/AIDS after completing treatment plan

Sexual Assault Prevention

- Incidence rate of sexual assault reported by females

Disabilities

- Percentage of newborns with neural tube defects
- Percentage of persons aged 18-65 with disabilities who are in the workforce
- Percentage of children aged 6 or younger with blood lead greater that 10 micrograms per deciliter[15]
- Percentage of women who gave birth in the past year and reported alcohol, tobacco, or other drugs during pregnancy

Emergency Medical Services

- Percentage of persons who suffer out-of-hospital cardiac arrest who survive

---

[12]Although the estimated incidence rate would be a more appropriate measure for monitoring progress by the state substance abuse agencies, the currently available data source for this measure provides prevalence data.

[13]See fn. 12.

[14]See fn. 12.

[15]See fn. 1.

POTENTIAL MEASURES

Measure Type:	**Chronic disease risk status**
Measure:	**Percentage of (a) persons aged 18-24 and (b) persons aged 25 and older currently smoking tobacco.**

Numerator:	All adults in each age group smoking tobacco (either statewide or in selected subgroups).
Denominator:	All adults in each age group (in the selected subgroup).
Rationale for Measure:	Use of smoking tobacco is the leading preventable cause of death in this country and a major cause of a wide range of chronic diseases. (This measure corresponds to *Healthy People 2000* Objective 3.4.)
Limitations of Measure:	Tobacco use by a state's population can be affected by many factors, including exposure to advertising, availability of vending machines, and other factors that may not be under the direct control of the state health agencies.
Use of Measure:	This outcome measure should be used in conjunction with relevant process and capacity measures in order to gain a sense of whether the actions taken by the state health agencies are having the desired impact.
Data Resources:	Behavioral Risk Factor Surveillance System (BRFSS).
Limitations of Data:	The methodology used to collect BRFSS data may vary significantly across states, making interstate comparisons with these data alone problematic.

Measure Type:	Chronic disease risk status
Measure:	Percentage of persons aged 14-17 (grades 9-12) currently smoking tobacco.

Numerator:	Young adults aged 14-17 currently smoking tobacco (either statewide or in selected sub-group).
Denominator:	Young adults aged 14-17 (in the selected sub-group).
Rationale for Measure:	Use of smoking tobacco is the leading prevent-able cause of death in this country and a major cause of a wide range of chronic diseases. Use generally begins during youth. (This measure corresponds to *Healthy People 2000* Objective 3.5.)
Limitations of Measure:	Tobacco use by a state's population can be affected by many factors, including exposure to advertising, availability of vending machines, and other factors that may not be under the direct control of the state health agencies. A school-based measure misses dropouts who may be at an increased risk for tobacco use, so supplemen-tal surveys of dropouts and absentees are needed for the most accurate measurement.
Use of Measure:	This outcome measure should be used in con-junction with relevant process and capacity measures in order to gain a sense of whether the actions taken by the state health agencies are having the desired impact.
Data Resources:	Youth Risk Behavior Surveillance System (YRBSS).
Limitations of Data:	The methodology used to collect YRBSS data may vary significantly across states, making interstate comparisons with these data alone problematic. It should also be noted that YRBSS is currently conducted in fewer than half of all states and often does not involve a representa-tive sampling of schools in a given state.

Measure Type:	**Chronic disease risk status**
Measure:	**Percentage of women who gave birth in the past year and reported smoking tobacco during pregnancy.**

Numerator:	All women who gave birth in the past year and reported smoking tobacco (either statewide or in selected subgroups).
Denominator:	All women giving birth (in selected subgroups).
Rationale for Measure:	Use of tobacco is the leading preventable cause of death in this country and a major cause of a wide range of chronic diseases. Use in pregnancy has deleterious effects on fetus and can raise the likelihood of one or more chronic diseases affecting the newborn. (This measure corresponds to *Healthy People 2000* Objective 14.10.)
Limitations of Measure:	Tobacco use by a state's childbearing-age female population can be affected by many factors, including exposure to advertising, availability of vending machines, and other factors that may not be under the direct control of the state health agencies.
Use of Measure:	This outcome measure should be used in conjunction with relevant process and capacity measures in order to gain a sense of whether the actions taken by the state health agencies are having the desired impact.
Data Resources:	
Numerator:	Birth certificate data; states with alternative methods for measuring tobacco use during pregnancy (for example, PRAMS) may opt to use these data instead.
Denominator:	Official state population estimate.
Limitations of Data:	It is widely understood that birth certificate data may understate the actual use of tobacco by pregnant women. Nevertheless, this should not be a problem in examining trends over time or making interstate comparisons if the reporting bias is consistent from one time period to another or across jurisdictions.

Measure Type:	Chronic disease risk status
Measure:	**Percentage of employed adults whose workplace has an official policy that bans smoking.**

Numerator:	All employed persons in worksites with tobacco policies (either statewide or in selected subgroups).
Denominator:	All employed persons (in selected subgroups).
Rationale for Measure:	Exposure to tobacco smoke by nonsmokers is a significant cause of chronic disease, including lung cancer.
Limitations of Measure:	Policies that limit tobacco use by a state's working population can be affected by many factors that may not be under the direct control of the state health agencies.
Use of Measure:	This outcome measure should be used in conjunction with relevant process and capacity measures in order to gain a sense of whether the actions taken by the state health agencies are having the desired impact.
Data Resources:	Current Population Survey (CPS), tobacco risk supplement.
Limitations of Data:	While the general CPS only provides state-level estimates for approximately ten states, data from the tobacco risk supplement to the CPS can be used to produce annual state level estimates for all states.

Measure Type:	**Chronic disease risk status**
Measure:	**Percentage of persons aged 18 and older who eat five or more servings of fruits and vegetables per day.***

Numerator:	Persons aged 18 and older who eat five or more servings of fruits and vegetables per day (either statewide or in selected subgroups).
Denominator:	All persons aged 18 and older (in the selected subgroup).
Rationale for Measure:	Eating five or more servings of fruits and vegetables per day is an important strategy for reducing dietary fat content, reducing obesity, and increasing the consumption of fiber and other nutrients, leading to reduced heart disease, colon cancer, and other diseases. (This measure corresponds to *Healthy People 2000* Objective 2.6.)
Limitations of Measure:	Although diet has been demonstrated to have a causal link in reducing heart disease and some cancers, other factors, such as heredity, are known to affect the incidence of these diseases.
Use of Measure:	This outcome measure should be used in conjunction with relevant process and capacity measures in order to gain a sense of whether the actions taken by the state health agencies are having the desired impact.
Data Resources:	Behavioral Risk Factor Surveillance System (BRFSS).
Limitations of Data:	The methodology used to collect BRFSS data may vary significantly across states, making interstate comparisons with these data alone problematic.

*The numerical value in this measure is the level that is generally regarded as appropriate by the medical community; it does not represent a level that has been independently determined or endorsed by the panel.

Measure Type:	**Chronic disease risk status**
Measure:	**Percentage of persons aged 14-17 (grades 9-12) who eat five or more servings of fruits and vegetables per day.***

Numerator:	Persons aged 14-17 who eat five or more servings of fruits and vegetables per day (either statewide or in selected subgroups).
Denominator:	All persons aged 14-17 (in the selected subgroup).
Rationale for Measure:	Eating five or more servings of fruits and vegetables per day is an important strategy for reducing dietary fat content, reducing obesity, and increasing the consumption of fiber and other nutrients, leading to reduced heart disease, colon cancer, and other diseases. Dietary habits may be established during childhood or adolescence. (This measure corresponds to *Healthy People 2000* Objective 2.6.)
Limitations of Measure:	Although diet has been demonstrated to have a causal link in reducing heart disease and some cancers, other factors, such as heredity, are known to affect the incidence of these diseases.
Use of Measure:	This outcome measure should be used in conjunction with relevant process and capacity measures in order to gain a sense of whether the actions taken by the state health agencies are having the desired impact.
Data Resources:	Youth Risk Behavior Surveillance System (YRBSS).
Limitations of Data:	The methodology used to collect YRBSS data may vary significantly across states, making interstate comparisons with these data alone problematic. It should also be noted that YRBSS is currently conducted in fewer than half of all states and often does not involve a representative sampling of schools in a given state.

*The numerical value in this measure is the level that is generally regarded as appropriate by the medical community; it does not represent a level that has been independently determined or endorsed by the panel.

Measure Type:	**Chronic disease risk status**
Measure:	**Percentage of persons aged 18 and older who are 20 percent or more above optimal body mass index.***

Numerator:	All persons aged 18 and older who are 20 percent or more above optimal body mass index (either statewide or in selected subgroups).
Denominator:	All persons aged 18 and older (in the selected subgroup).
Rationale for Measure:	Obesity is a proxy measure for excess total calorie intake and insufficient exercise, an important cause of chronic disease.
Limitations of Measure:	Although diet and exercise have been demonstrated to have a causal link in reducing heart disease and some cancers, other factors, such as heredity, are known to affect the incidence of these diseases.
Use of Measure:	This outcome measure should be used in conjunction with relevant process and capacity measures in order to gain a sense of whether the actions taken by the state health agencies are having the desired impact.
Data Resources:	Behavioral Risk Factor Surveillance System (BRFSS).
Limitations of Data:	The methodology used to collect BRFSS data may vary significantly across states, making interstate comparisons with these data alone problematic.

*The numerical value in this measure is the level that is generally regarded as appropriate by the medical community; it does not represent a level that has been independently determined or endorsed by the panel.

Measure Type:	Chronic disease risk status
Measure:	**Percentage of persons aged 18 and older who do not engage in physical activity or exercise**

Numerator:	Adults who do not engage in physical activity or exercise (either statewide or in selected subgroups).
Denominator:	All adults (in the selected subgroup).
Rationale for Measure:	Physical activity is a key determinant of overall wellness, and it reduces the risk of cardiovascular disease. (This measure corresponds to *Healthy People 2000* Objective 1.3.)
Limitations of Measure:	Although exercise has been demonstrated to have a causal link in reducing heart disease and some cancers, other factors, such as heredity, are known to affect the incidence of these diseases.
Use of Measure:	This outcome measure should be used in conjunction with relevant process and capacity measures in order to gain a sense of whether the actions taken by the state health agencies are having the desired impact.
Data Resources:	Behavioral Risk Factor Surveillance System (BRFSS).
Limitations of Data:	The methodology used to collect BRFSS data may vary significantly across states, making interstate comparisons with these data alone problematic.

Measure Type:	**Chronic disease risk status**
Measure:	**Percentage of persons aged 14-17 (grades 9-12) who do not engage in physical activity or exercise**
Numerator:	Persons aged 14-17 who do not engage in physical activity or exercise (either statewide or in selected subgroups).
Denominator:	All persons aged 14-17 (in the selected sub-group).
Rationale for Measure:	Physical activity is a key determinant of overall wellness, and it reduces the risk of cardiovascular disease. Exercise habits may be established during childhood or adolescence. (This measure corresponds to *Healthy People 2000* Objective 1.3.)
Limitations of Measure:	Although exercise has been demonstrated to have a causal link in reducing heart disease and some cancers, other factors, such as heredity, are known to affect the incidence of these diseases.
Use of Measure:	This outcome measure should be used in conjunction with relevant process and capacity measures in order to gain a sense of whether the actions taken by the state health agencies are having the desired impact.
Data Resources:	Youth Risk Behavior Surveillance System (YRBSS).
Limitations of Data:	The methodology used to collect YRBSS data may vary significantly across states, making interstate comparisons with these data alone problematic. It should also be noted that YRBSS is currently conducted in fewer than half of all states and often does not involve a representative sampling of schools in a given state.

Measure Type:	**Chronic disease risk status**
Measure:	**Percentage of persons aged 18 and older who had their blood pressure checked within past 2 years.***

Numerator:	Persons 18 and older having blood pressure checked within past 2 years (either statewide or in selected subgroups)
Denominator:	All persons 18 and older (in selected subgroups).
Rationale for Measure:	Hypertension is a key determinant of cardiovascular and cerebrovascular disease. A key public health component of prevention is screening. (This measure corresponds to *Healthy People 2000* Objective 15.13.)
Limitations of Measure:	While decreasing hypertension has been shown to be a way of improving cardiovascular and cerebrovascular functioning, other factors are known to influence the incidence of cardiovascular and cerebrovascular disease.
Use of Measure:	This outcome measure should be used in conjunction with relevant process and capacity measures in order to gain a sense of whether the actions taken by the state health agencies are having the desired impact.
Data Resources:	Behavioral Risk Factor Surveillance System (BRFSS).
Limitations of Data:	The methodology used to collect BRFSS data may vary significantly across states, making interstate comparisons with these data alone problematic.

---

*The numerical value in this measure is the level that is generally regarded as appropriate by the medical community; it does not represent a level that has been independently determined or endorsed by the panel.

Measure Type:	**Chronic disease risk status**
Measure:	**Percentage of women aged 45 and older and men aged 35 and older who had their cholesterol checked within past 5 years.***
Numerator:	Persons 18 and older having cholesterol checked within past 5 years (either statewide or in selected subgroups).
Denominator:	All persons 18 and older (in selected subgroups).
Rationale for Measure:	Hypercholesterolemia is a key determinant of cardiovascular disease. A key public health component of prevention is screening. (This measure corresponds to *Healthy People 2000* Objective 15.14.)
Limitations of Measure:	While decreasing hypercholesterolemia has been shown to improve cardiovascular functioning, other factors are known to influence the incidence of cardiovascular disease.
Use of Measure:	This outcome measure should be used in conjunction with relevant process and capacity measures in order to gain a sense of whether the actions taken by the state health agencies are having the desired impact.
Data Resources:	Behavioral Risk Factor Surveillance System (BRFSS).
Limitations of Data:	The methodology used to collect BRFSS data may vary significantly across states, making interstate comparisons with these data alone problematic.

---

*The numerical value in this measure is the level that is generally regarded as appropriate by the medical community; it does not represent a level that has been independently determined or endorsed by the panel.

Measure Type:	**Chronic disease risk status**
Measure:	**Percentage of women aged 50 and older who received a mammogram within past 2 years.***

Numerator:	Women aged 50 and older who received a mammogram within the previous two years (either statewide or in selected subgroups).
Denominator:	All women aged 50 and older (in selected subgroups).
Rationale for Measure:	Mammography is a primary strategy for early detection and thus more favorable treatment outcome for breast cancer. (This measure corresponds to *Healthy People 2000* Objective 16.11.)
Limitations of Measure:	While early detection and treatment have been shown to improve outcomes for breast cancer, other factors can also influence mortality from this disease.
Use of Measure:	This outcome measure should be used in conjunction with relevant process and capacity measures in order to gain a sense of whether the actions taken by the state health agencies are having the desired impact.
Data Resources:	Behavioral Risk Factor Surveillance System (BRFSS).
Limitations of Data:	The methodology used to collect BRFSS data may vary significantly across states, making interstate comparisons with these data alone problematic.

---

*The numerical value in this measure is the level that is generally regarded as appropriate by the medical community; it does not represent a level that has been independently determined or endorsed by the panel. Breast cancer incidence by diagnosed stage may be a better alternative in cancer registry areas; this would be a health status outcome measure.

Measure Type:	Chronic disease risk status
Measure:	**Percentage of adults aged 50 and older who had a fecal occult blood test within past 12 months or a flexible sigmoidoscopy within past 5 years.***

Numerator:	Adults aged 50 and older who have had a fecal occult blood test within past 12 months or a flexible sigmoidoscopy within past 5 years (either statewide or in selected subgroups).
Denominator:	All adults aged 50 and older (in the selected subgroup).
Rationale for Measure:	Fecal occult blood testing or periodic sigmoidoscopy are primary strategies for early detection and thus more favorable treatment outcome for colon cancer. (This measure corresponds to *Healthy People 2000* Objective 16.13.)
Limitations of Measure:	While early detection has been shown to improve treatment outcomes for colon cancer, other factors can also influence the mortality of this disease.
Use of Measure:	This outcome measure should be used in conjunction with relevant process and capacity measures in order to gain a sense of whether the actions taken by the state health agencies are having the desired impact.
Data Resources:	Behavioral Risk Factor Surveillance System (BRFSS).
Limitations of Data:	The methodology used to collect BRFSS data may vary significantly across states, making interstate comparisons with these data alone problematic.

*The numerical value in this measure is the level that is generally regarded as appropriate by the medical community; it does not represent a level that has been independently determined or endorsed by the panel. Colon cancer incidence by diagnosed stage may be a better alternative in cancer registry areas; this would be a health status outcome measure.

Measure Type:	**Chronic disease risk status**
Measure:	**Percentage of women aged 18 and older who received a Pap smear within past 3 years.***

Numerator:	Women aged 18 and older who received a Pap smear within past 3 years (either statewide or in selected subgroups).
Denominator:	All women aged 18 and older (in selected subgroups).
Rationale for Measure:	Pap smears are a primary strategy for early detection and thus more favorable treatment outcome for cervical cancer. (This measure corresponds to *Healthy People 2000* Objective 16.12.)
Limitations of Measure:	While early detection and treatment have been shown to improve outcomes for cervical cancer, other factors can also influence mortality from this disease.
Use of Measure:	This outcome measure should be used in conjunction with relevant process and capacity measures in order to gain a sense of whether the actions taken by the state health agencies are having the desired impact.
Data Resources:	Behavioral Risk Factor Surveillance System (BRFSS).
Limitations of Data:	The methodology used to collect BRFSS data may vary significantly across states, making interstate comparisons with these data alone problematic.

---

*The numerical value in this measure is the level that is generally regarded as appropriate by the medical community; it does not represent a level that has been independently determined or endorsed by the panel. Invasive cervical cancer incidence by diagnosed stage is a better alternative in cancer registry areas; this would be a health status outcome measure.

Measure Type:	Chronic disease risk status
Measure:	Percentage of persons with diabetes who had HbA1C checked within past 12 months.*

Numerator:	Adult diabetics who receive HbA1C screening at least annually (either statewide or in selected subgroups).
Denominator:	All adult diabetics (in the selected subgroup).
Rationale for Measure:	HbA1C is a measure of blood glucose control. Good control of blood glucose has been shown to prevent secondary complications of diabetes. Routine testing of HbA1C can identify diabetics who need additional intervention to achieve optimal control.
Limitations of Measure:	While early detection of problems in controlling blood glucose levels has been shown to improve treatment outcomes for diabetes, other factors can also influence the morbidity and mortality caused by this disease.
Use of Measure:	This outcome measure should be used in conjunction with relevant process and capacity measures in order to gain a sense of whether the actions taken by the state health agencies are having the desired impact.
Data Resources:	Behavioral Risk Factor Surveillance System (BRFSS); Medicare Statistical Data System.
Limitations of Data:	The sample of diabetics identified through the BRFSS may be too small to obtain accurate estimates of those receiving HbA1C screening. Also, the methodology used to collect BRFSS data may vary significantly across states, making interstate comparisons problematic. The Medicare population within the Medicare Statistical Data System is not representative of all diabetics, and it may not be representative of the Medicare diabetic population in some areas as it does not include encounter information from Medicare managed care services.

*The numerical value in this measure is the level that is generally regarded as appropriate by the medical community; it does not represent a level that has been independently determined or endorsed by the panel.

Measure Type:	**Chronic disease risk status**
Measure:	**Percentage of persons with diabetes who had a health professional examine their feet at least once within past 12 months.***

Numerator:	Adult diabetics who have received a foot exam within past 12 months (either statewide or in selected subgroups).
Denominator:	All adult diabetics (in selected subgroups).
Rationale for Measure:	Diabetics are at risk for peripheral vascular disease and lower extremity amputation. Routine foot exams can identify at-risk patients early and lead to improved outcomes.
Limitations of Measure:	While early detection of circulatory problems has been shown to improve treatment outcomes for diabetes, other factors can also influence the morbidity and mortality caused by this disease.
Use of Measure:	This outcome measure should be used in conjunction with relevant process and capacity measures in order to gain a sense of whether the actions taken by the state health agencies are having the desired impact.
Data Resources:	Behavioral Risk Factor Surveillance System (BRFSS); Medicare Statistical Data System.
Limitations of Data:	The sample of diabetics identified through the BRFSS may be too small to obtain accurate estimates of those receiving HbA1C screening. Also, the methodology used to collect BRFSS data may vary significantly across states, making interstate comparisons with these data alone problematic. The Medicare population within the Medicare Statistical Data System is not representative of all diabetics, and may not be representative of the Medicare diabetic population in some areas as it does not include encounter information from Medicare managed care services.

*The numerical value in this measure is the level that is generally regarded as appropriate by the medical community; it does not represent a level that has been independently determined or endorsed by the panel.

Measure Type:	**Chronic disease risk status**
Measure:	**Percentage of persons with diabetes who received a dilated eye exam within past 12 months.***

Numerator:	Adult diabetics who have received an eye exam in the past year (either statewide or in selected subgroups).
Denominator:	All adult diabetics (in the selected subgroup).
Rationale for Measure:	Diabetics are at risk for diabetic retinopathy and blindness. Routine eye exams can identify at-risk patients early and lead to improved outcomes. (This measure corresponds to *Healthy People 2000* Objective 17.23.)
Limitations of Measure:	While early detection has been shown to improve treatment outcomes for diabetes, other factors can also influence the morbidity and mortality caused by this disease.
Use of Measure:	This outcome measure should be used in conjunction with relevant process and capacity measures in order to gain a sense of whether the actions taken by the state health agencies are having the desired impact.
Data Resources:	Behavioral Risk Factor Surveillance System (BRFSS); Medicare Statistical Data System.
Limitations of Data:	The sample of diabetics identified through the BRFSS may be too small to obtain accurate estimates of those receiving HbA1C screening. Also, the methodology used to collect BRFSS data may vary significantly across states, making interstate comparisons with these data alone problematic. The Medicare population within the Medicare Statistical Data System is not representative of all diabetics, and may not be representative of the Medicare diabetic population in some areas as it does not include encounter information from Medicare managed care services.

---

*The numerical value in this measure is the level that is generally regarded as appropriate by the medical community; it does not represent a level that has been independently determined or endorsed by the panel.

Measure Type:	STD health status outcome
Measure:	Incidence rates of selected STDs: gonococcal urethritis in men; chlamydial urethritis in men; primary and secondary syphilis; congenital syphilis.

Numerator:	Number of reported cases.
Denominator:	Official state population estimates.
Rationale for Measure:	Used by CDC, states, and localities to track health status and overall STD prevention efforts. This is a useful measure because treatment of early acute conditions prevents the spread of new infections.
Limitations of Measure:	Useful information is limited to segments of the community whose health providers systematically report disease. Measure does not capture information from nonreporting sectors nor does it distinguish between cases from high-transmitting core groups and those from other groups. Factors other than program effects, such as poverty, health access, and substance abuse influence incidence. Variation in reported rates may be due to changes in the intensity of health department case finding and screening activities, rather than to true changes in disease incidence.
Use of Measure:	Disease specific measures of incidence have specific value in evaluating programs focused on these diseases. Changes in multiple incidence measures can be used to assess broader prevention efforts, e.g., those aimed at risk reduction or improving access to services. These outcome measures should be used in conjunction with relevant process and capacity measures in order to gain a sense of whether the actions taken by the state health agencies are having the desired impact.
Data Resources:	National, state, and local STD surveillance systems.
Limitations of Data:	There is substantial variability in the diagnostic laboratory testing and reporting practices of providers. Shifts in populations at risk served by providers may not be reported in a timely manner because of this variability.

Measure Type:	HIV health status outcome
Measure:	Incidence rates of HIV infection: newly diagnosed cases of HIV infection; perinatally acquired HIV infection of infants.

Numerator:	Number of newly diagnosed cases of HIV infection in selected subgroups.
Denominator:	Official state population estimates.
Rationale for Measure:	Used by some states as a proxy measure for the occurrence of new HIV infection. Reducing new infection is the goal of prevention programs.
Limitations of Measure:	Useful information is limited to segments of the community whose health providers systematically report disease. The actual onset of the infection is not measured by this indicator; rather, the measure depends on screening frequencies, access to services, and trust between people and their providers. Many factors other than program activities influence new infection rates, including poverty, discrimination, and injection drug use.
Use of Measure:	Trends in the incidence of HIV infections are useful in measuring prevention efforts. This outcome measure should be used in conjunction with relevant process and capacity measures in order to gain a sense of whether the actions taken by the state health agencies are having the desired impact.
Data Resources:	State-based HIV reporting systems.
Limitations of Data:	HIV reporting systems are available only in some states. Rates of diagnosis depend heavily on the level of case finding through screening. The selection of providers by at-risk populations may be influenced by the perceived likelihood of provider reporting. Major changes in HIV treatment and diagnostic criteria may influence the enumeration of cases.

Measure Type:	STD health status outcome
Measure:	Prevalence rates of selected STDs: gonococcal infection in women in defined populations; genital chlamydial infection in defined populations; syphilis in defined risk groups, e.g., pregnant women; rectal gonococcal infection in men.

Numerator:	Reported number of existing infections at specific monitoring site.
Denominator:	Population attending specific monitoring site.
Rationale for Measure:	Prevalent cases are the source of new infections in a community. Reducing the duration of prevalent infections contributes to STD prevention.
Limitations of Measure:	Monitoring is established only at defined sites, and the use of those sites by populations at risk will vary over time and location. The validity and reliability of the measure is dependent on the quality of the laboratory procedures.
Use of Measure:	Consistent trends in prevalence in well-defined populations, particularly when monitored at multiple locations in a state, can provide a reasonable estimate of whether true prevalence is changing. When used in conjunction with relevant process and capacity measures, the measure can assist in determining whether a state effort is having the desired impact.
Data Resources:	Special state-based programmatic surveys; publicly supported screening programs; Regional Infertility Prevention Project; several state and local STD programs.
Limitations of Data:	For a given state, the generalizability of data depends on the number of monitoring sites, how they are selected, and consistent assurance that either a complete or systematic sample is obtained at each site. Variations in these data collection procedures make cross-state comparisons problematic.

Measure Type:	HIV health status outcome
Measure:	Prevalence rates of HIV infection: seroprevalence of HIV infection in defined populations at high risk of infection, e.g., women of childbearing age.

Numerator:	Reported number of existing infections.
Denominator:	Populations attending specific monitoring site.
Rationale for Measure:	Prevalent cases are the source of new infections in a community.
Limitations of Measure:	Monitoring is established only at defined sites, and the use of those sites by populations at risk will vary over time and location. The validity and reliability of the measure is dependent on the quality of laboratory procedures.
Use of Measure:	Consistent trends in prevalence in well-defined populations, particularly when monitored at multiple locations in a state, can provide a reasonable estimate of whether true prevalence is changing. When used in conjunction with relevant process and capacity measures, the measure can assist in determining whether a state effort is having the desired impact.
Data Resources:	Special state-based programmatic surveys.
Limitations of Data:	For a given state, the generalizability of data depends on the number of monitoring sites, how they are selected, and consistent assurance that either a complete or systematic sample is obtained at each site. Variations in these data collection procedures make cross-state comparisons problematic.

Measure Type:	STD, HIV infection, and tuberculosis consumer satisfaction
Measure:	**Rate of consumer satisfaction with STD, HIV infection, and tuberculosis treatment programs: satisfaction with (a) access to services; (b) appropriateness of services; and (c) perceptions of gain in personal outcomes.**

Numerator:	Number of persons served by STD/HIV/TB clinical services satisfied with access and appropriateness of services and gain in personal outcomes.
Denominator:	All persons who use STD/HIV/TB services.
Rationale for Measure:	Satisfaction of the person who uses STD/HIV/TB clinical services is a critical measure of the viability of prevention programs. If consumers are not satisfied with services, they may not use services.
Limitations of Measure:	Variations in consumer satisfaction surveys across states make interstate comparisons problematic.
Use of Measure:	This outcome measure should be used in conjunction with relevant process and capacity measures in order to gain a sense of whether the actions taken by the state health agencies are having the desired impact.
Data Resources:	Special state surveys.
Limitations of Data:	Obtaining satisfaction surveys from the broad range of clinical providers is problematic. It is particularly difficult to assess consumer satisfaction among people who use services only episodically.

Measure Type:	**STD and HIV risk status**
Measure:	**Rates of sexual activity among adolescents aged 14-17.**
Numerator:	Number of sexually active adolescents who have engaged in sexual intercourse during the past 3 months.
Denominator:	Number of adolescents in population.
Rationale for Measure:	Once a person has become sexually active there are two definite actions they can take to reduce the risk of contracting STDs or HIV infection: abstain or reduce the frequency of sexual intercourse. (This measure corresponds to *Healthy People 2000* Objective 5.5.)
Limitations of Measure:	Although high rates of sexual activity can increase the risk of contracting STDs or HIV, this measure does not take into account other factors that may play a role, including frequency of sexual activity, number of partners, and protection methods used.
Use of Measure:	This outcome measure should be used in conjunction with relevant process and capacity measures in order to gain a sense of whether the actions taken by the state health agencies are having the desired impact.
Data Resources:	The Youth Risk Behavior Surveillance System (YRBSS) and other state-based population surveys.
Limitations of Data:	The methodology used to collect such data may vary significantly across states, making interstate comparisons problematic. The YRBSS is currently conducted in fewer than half of all states and often does not involve a representative sampling of schools in a given state. It also does not capture information about adolescents who are not attending school.

Measure Type:	**STD and HIV risk status**
Measure:	**Rates of sexual activity with multiple sex partners among people aged 18 and older.**

Numerator:	Number of persons aged 18 and older who have engaged in sexual intercourse with more than one partner during the past 12 months.
Denominator:	Number of persons aged 18 and older in the population who have ever been sexually active.
Rationale for Measure:	Once a person has become sexually active there are two definite actions they can take to reduce the risk of contracting STDs or HIV infection: abstain or reduce the frequency of sexual intercourse. (This measure corresponds to *Healthy People 2000* Objective 5.5.)
Limitations of Measure:	Although high rates of sexual activity can increase the risk of contracting STDs or HIV, this measure does not take into account other factors that may play a role, including frequency of sexual activity, number of partners, and protection methods used.
Use of Measure:	This outcome measure should be used in conjunction with relevant process and capacity measures in order to gain a sense of whether the actions taken by the state health agencies are having the desired impact.
Data Resources:	The Behavior Risk Factor Surveillance System (BRFSS) and other state-based population surveys.
Limitations of Data:	The methodology used to collect such data may vary significantly across states, making interstate comparisons problematic. BRFSS may not contain a sufficient sample of the high risk group of interest, unless states using this measure supplement the sample.

Measure Type:	STD and HIV risk status
Measure:	Rates of condom use during last episode of sexual intercourse among sexually active adolescents aged 14-17.

Numerator:	Number of sexually active adolescents aged 14-17 who used condoms during their last episode of sexual intercourse.
Denominator:	Number of adolescents aged 14-17 who have ever engaged in sexual intercourse.
Rationale for Measure:	If adolescents engage in sexual intercourse, the use of condoms reduces the likelihood of contracting or spreading HIV or STDs. (This measure corresponds to *Healthy People 2000* Objective 5.6 for people aged 19 and younger.)
Limitations of Measure:	Although the use of condoms reduces the likelihood of contracting or spreading STDs or HIV, a person's behavior during the most recent episode of sexual intercourse may not be representative of regular behavior.
Use of Measure:	This outcome measure should be used in conjunction with relevant process and capacity measures in order to gain a sense of whether the actions taken by the state health agencies are having the desired impact.
Data Resources:	The Youth Risk Behavior Surveillance System (YRBSS) and other state-based population surveys.
Limitations of Data:	The methodology used to collect such data may vary significantly across states, making interstate comparisons problematic. The YRBSS is currently conducted in fewer than half of all states and often does not involve a representative sampling of schools in a given state. It also does not capture information about adolescents who are not attending school.

Measure Type:	**STD and HIV risk status**
Measure:	**Rates of condom use by persons aged 18 and older with multiple sex partners during last episode of sexual intercourse.**

Numerator:	Number of persons aged 18 and older with multiple sex partners who used condoms during their last episode of sexual intercourse.
Denominator:	Number of persons aged 18 and older with multiple sex partners
Rationale for Measure:	Persons who engage in sexual intercourse with multiple partners are at increased risk of contracting or spreading STDs or HIV infection; the use of condoms reduces this risk. (This measure corresponds to *Healthy People 2000* Objective 5.6 for people aged 19 and younger.)
Limitations of Measure:	Although the use of condoms reduces the likelihood of contracting or spreading STDs or HIV, a person's behavior during the most recent episode of sexual intercourse may not be representative of regular behavior.
Use of Measure:	This outcome measure should be used in conjunction with relevant process and capacity measures in order to gain a sense of whether the actions taken by the state health agencies are having the desired impact.
Data Resources:	The Behavior Risk Factor Surveillance System (BRFSS) and other state-based population surveys.
Limitations of Data:	The methodology used to collect such data may vary significantly across states, making interstate comparisons problematic. BRFSS may not contain a sufficient sample of the high risk group of interest, unless states using this measure supplement the sample.

Measure Type:	STD and HIV risk status
Measure:	**Rates of condom use during last episode of sexual intercourse among men having sex with men.**

Numerator:	Number of men who have sex with men who used condoms during their last episode of sexual intercourse.
Denominator:	Number of men who have sex with men who have ever engaged in sexual intercourse.
Rationale for Measure:	The use of condoms reduces the likelihood of contracting or spreading HIV or STDs. (This measure corresponds to *Healthy People 2000* Objective 5.6 for people aged 19 and younger.)
Limitations of Measure:	Although the use of condoms reduces the likelihood of contracting or spreading STDs or HIV, a person's behavior during the most recent episode of sexual intercourse may not be representative of regular behavior.
Use of Measure:	This outcome measure should be used in conjunction with relevant process and capacity measures in order to gain a sense of whether the actions taken by the state health agencies are having the desired impact.
Data Resources:	The Behavior Risk Factor Surveillance System (BRFSS) and other state-based population surveys.
Limitations of Data:	The methodology used to collect such data may vary significantly across states, making interstate comparisons problematic. BRFSS may not contain a sufficient sample of the high risk group of interest, unless states using this measure supplement the sample.

Measure Type:	**HIV/AIDS risk status**
Measure:	**Rates of injection drug use among adolescents and adults.**

Numerator:	Number of adolescents and adults who have engaged in injection drug use.
Denominator:	Number of adolescents and adults.
Rationale for Measure:	A major known contributor to the transmission of HIV/AIDS is injection drug use. Because of the long time between exposure and onset of AIDS, it is recommended that states monitor the proportion of the population engaged in injection drug use.
Limitations of Measure:	This measure provides only a crude estimate of the frequency of injection drug use (i.e., past year for adults and any time in the past for adolescents).
Use of Measure:	This outcome measure should be used in conjunction with relevant process and capacity measures in order to gain a sense of whether the actions taken by the state health agencies are having the desired impact.
Data Resources:	The Behavior Risk Factor Surveillance System (BRFSS), the Youth Risk Behavior Surveillance System (YRBSS), and other state-based population surveys.
Limitations of Data:	The methodology used to collect such data may vary significantly across states, making interstate comparisons problematic. BRFSS and YRBSS may not contain a sufficient sample of the high risk group of interest, unless states using this measure supplement the sample. This is especially true for the YRBSS which is currently conducted in fewer than half of all states and often does not involve a representative sampling of schools in a given state.

Measure Type:	STD, HIV, and tuberculosis risk status
Measure:	**Completion rates of treatment for STDs, HIV infection, and tuberculosis: standard treatment of individuals with STDs and their sex partners; standard antiviral treatment of HIV-infected pregnant women and their infants; standard treatment of tuberculosis cases, contacts, and skin test converters.**
Numerator:	Number of cases of prescribed treatment completion for each disease.
Denominator:	Total number of cases of prescribed treatment for each disease.
Rationale for Measure:	Adequate treatment of curable infections is a primary strategy to prevent further spread in a community. There is direct evidence that adequate treatment directly reduces the risk of infection to others.
Limitations of Measure:	Treatment of cases in populations of high transmitters is more beneficial than the treatment of noncore groups.
Use of Measure:	The measure, when used in conjunction with measures of incidence and prevalence and the other relevant process and capacity measures, can be a useful measure of risk status in the community.
Data Resources:	State-specific treatment surveys.
Limitations of Data:	Treatment is poorly documented in some medical records. Whether data are collected depends on the existence of some form of disease reporting system or registry. Available data are likely to be biased toward higher rates of adequate treatment because sex partners not identified by the index patient, the provider, or the health department may be less likely to receive adequate treatment.

Measure Type:	**Mental health status outcome**
Measure:	**Percentage of persons aged 18 and older receiving mental health services who experience reduced psychological distress.**

Numerator:	Change in psychological distress from beginning treatment to discharge.
Denominator:	Number of persons aged 18 and older admitted for services and then discharged.
Rationale for Measure:	Psychological distress (or symptom reduction) is one of the most widely accepted methods of evaluating the impact of mental health services.
Limitations of Measure:	Variations in assessment mechanisms across states make interstate comparisons problematic.
Use of Measure:	This outcome measure should be used in conjunction with relevant process and capacity measures in order to gain a sense of whether the actions taken by the state agencies are having the desired impact.
Data Resources:	
Numerator:	Consumer or provider surveys, using one or more of the following instruments: NYCMH, Basis 32, SF 36, Multnomah Community Ability Scale, and Lehman Quality of Life.
Denominator:	State data systems.
Limitations of Data:	Surveys are not available in many states, and where available may be limited by numerous sources of error: e.g., coverage error, which is the result of neglecting to measure all parts of the population; nonresponse error, which is caused by individuals who refuse the survey or cannot be located; and sampling error, which reflects the difference between the general population and the specific sample chosen for the survey.

Measure Type:	Mental health social functioning
Measure:	Percentage of persons aged 18 and older receiving mental health services who experience increased level of functioning.

Numerator:	Change in level of functioning from beginning treatment to discharge.
Denominator:	Number of persons aged 18 and older admitted for services and then discharged.
Rationale for Measure:	Increase in functioning is one of the most important means of determining whether positive change has occurred.
Limitations of Measure:	Variations in surveys across states make interstate comparisons problematic.
Use of Measure:	This outcome measure should be used in conjunction with relevant process and capacity measures in order to gain a sense of whether the actions taken by the state agencies are having the desired impact.
Data Resources:	
Numerator:	Consumer or provider surveys using one or more of the following instruments: CAR, FARS, NYLOC.
Denominator:	State data systems.
Limitations of Data:	Surveys are not available in many states, and where available may be limited by numerous sources of error: e.g., coverage error, which is the result of neglecting to measure all parts of the population; nonresponse error, which is caused by individuals who refuse the survey or cannot be located; and sampling error, which reflects the difference between the general population and the specific sample chosen for the survey.

Measure Type:	**Mental health social functioning**
Measure:	**Percentage of persons aged 18 and older receiving mental health services who report increased employment (including volunteer time).**

Numerator:	Number of consumers aged 18 and older reporting increased employment.
Denominator:	Total number of consumers aged 18 and older.
Rationale for Measure:	Consumers, providers, and funders consistently identify employment as one of the most critical measures of program success.
Limitations of Measure:	Variations in surveys across states make interstate comparisons problematic.
Use of Measure:	This outcome measure should be used in conjunction with relevant process and capacity measures in order to gain a sense of whether the actions taken by the state agencies are having the desired impact.
Data Resources:	
Numerator:	Consumer surveys.
Denominator:	State data systems.
Limitations of Data:	Surveys are not available in many states, and where available may be limited by numerous sources of error: e.g., coverage error, which is the result of neglecting to measure all parts of the population; nonresponse error, which is caused by individuals who refuse the survey or cannot be located; and sampling error, which reflects the difference between the general population and the specific sample chosen for the survey.

Measure Type:	Mental health social functioning
Measure:	Percentage of persons aged 18 and older with serious and persistent mental illness receiving mental health services who live in integrated, independent living situations or with family members.

Numerator:	All consumers aged 18 and older with serious and persistent mental illness who live in integrated, independent living situations or with family members.
Denominator:	All consumers aged 18 and older with serious and persistent mental illness.
Rationale for Measure:	Integrated, independent living or living with family members is the goal of many funding agencies and most consumers.
Limitations of Measure:	Significant variation in quality of living situations may occur among consumers living independently or with family members.
Use of Measure:	This outcome measure should be used in conjunction with relevant process and capacity measures in order to gain a sense of whether the actions taken by the state agencies are having the desired impact.
Data Resources:	State data systems.
Limitations of Data:	Surveys are not available in many states, and where available may be limited by numerous sources of error: e.g., coverage error, which is the result of neglecting to measure all parts of the population; nonresponse error, which is caused by individuals who refuse the survey or cannot be located; and sampling error, which reflects the difference between the general population and the specific sample chosen for the survey.

Measure Type:	Mental health social functioning
Measure:	Percentage of children aged 17 and younger with serious emotional disorders receiving mental health services who live in noncustodial living situations.

Numerator:	Number of children aged 17 and younger with serious emotional disorders who are not in out-of-home placement.
Denominator:	Number of children aged 17 and younger with serious emotional disorders.
Rationale for Measure:	Some children need to be in out-of-home placements. However, many states identify a goal of reducing out-of-home placements as a measure of success of the mental health programs.
Limitations of Measure:	Significant variation in quality of living situations may occur among consumers in noncustodial living situations.
Use of Measure:	This outcome measure should be used in conjunction with relevant process and capacity measures in order to gain a sense of whether the actions taken by state agencies are having the desired impact.
Data Resources	
Numerator:	State mental health data systems; Medicaid data; child welfare data; juvenile justice data.
Denominator:	State mental health data system.
Limitations of Data:	Surveys are not available in many states, and where available may be limited by numerous sources of error: e.g., coverage error, which is the result of neglecting to measure all parts of the population; nonresponse error, which is caused by individuals who refuse the survey or cannot be located; and sampling error, which reflects the difference between the general population and the specific sample chosen for the survey.

Measure Type:	Mental health social functioning
Measure:	Percentage of persons aged 18 and older with serious mental illness who are in prisons and jails.

Numerator:	Number of adults aged 18 and older with serious mental illness in jails and prisons.
Denominator:	Number of adults aged 18 and older with serious mental illness.
Rationale for Measure:	The number of adults with serious mental illness in jails and prisons is increasing. While some individuals with serious mental illness are appropriately in jails and prisons, others are there because there is no other facility providing services.
Limitations of Measure:	In many states the mental health agency does not have the responsibility for delivering or administering services to the jail and prison population. The measure can be affected by many factors that may not be under the direct control of the mental health agencies.
Use of Measure:	This outcome measure should be used in conjunction with relevant process and capacity measures in order to gain a sense of whether the actions taken by the state agencies are having the desired impact.
Data Resources:	State corrections data sets; state surveys of mentally ill persons.
Limitations of Data:	There are difficulties in obtaining valid and reliable data on prison and jail populations. The methodology required to accurately and meaningfully measure this subpopulation is not widely available or developed. In addition, it may be hard to obtain information on jails and prisons, and it is often difficult to coordinate data across agencies.

Measure Type:	Mental health social functioning
Measure:	Percentage of children aged 17 and younger with serious emotional disorders who are in juvenile justice facilities.

Numerator:	Number of children aged 17 and younger with serious emotional disorders who are in juvenile justice facilities.
Denominator:	Number of children aged 17 and younger with serious emotional disorders.
Rationale for Measure:	Many states identify a goal of reducing the number in juvenile justice facilities as a measure of success of mental health programs.
Limitations of Measure:	In many states the mental health agency does not have responsibility for delivering or administering services to the juvenile justice facility population. The measure can be affected by many factors that may not be under the direct control of the mental health agencies.
Use of Measure:	This outcome measure should be used in conjunction with relevant process and capacity measures in order to gain a sense of whether the actions taken by the state agencies are having the desired impact.
Data Resources:	
Numerator:	State data systems; child welfare and juvenile justice.
Denominator:	State data system.
Limitations of Data:	There are difficulties in obtaining valid and reliable data on juvenile justice facility populations. The methodology required to accurately and meaningfully measure this subpopulation is not widely available or developed.

Measure Type:	**Mental health social functioning**
Measure:	**Percentage of homeless persons aged 18 and older who have a serious mental illness.**
Numerator:	Number of persons aged 18 and older with serious mental illness who are homeless.
Denominator:	Number of persons aged 18 and older who are homeless.
Rationale for Measure:	Homelessness is one of the most serious problems for many people with serious mental illness.
Limitations of Measure:	In many states the mental health agency does not have the responsibility for delivering or administering services to the homeless population. The measure can be affected by many factors that may not be under the direct control of the mental health agencies.
Use of Measure:	This outcome measure should be used in conjunction with relevant process and capacity measures in order to gain a sense of whether the actions taken by the state agencies are having the desired impact.
Data Resources:	
Numerator:	Estimates of homeless populations from local surveys and shelter information.
Denominator:	State surveys of population-in-need estimates, based on new federal definitions.
Limitations of Data:	There are difficulties in obtaining valid and reliable data on the homeless population. The methodology required to accurately and meaningfully measure this subpopulation is not widely available or developed. In addition, it is nearly impossible to collect data on the homeless if they do not reach a shelter. These data are not available in many states.

Measure Type:	**Mental health consumer satisfaction**
Measure:	**Percentage of adolescents aged 14-17 or family members of children and adolescents or both who are satisfied with: (a) access to services, (b) appropriateness of services, and (c) perceptions of gain in personal outcomes.**

Numerator:	All adolescents aged 14-17 or family members of children and adolescents or both who are surveyed and are satisfied with access to and appropriateness of services and gain in personal outcomes.
Denominator:	All adolescents aged 14-17 or family members surveyed or both who use services.
Rationale for Measure:	Satisfaction of the person using mental health services is a critical measure of the viability of service programs. If consumers are not satisfied with services, they may not use them.
Limitations of Measure:	Variations in consumer satisfaction surveys across states make interstate comparisons problematic.
Use of Measure:	This outcome measure should be used in conjunction with relevant process and capacity measures in order to gain a sense of whether the actions taken by the state agencies are having the desired impact.
Data Resources:	MHSIP Report Card Survey; state surveys.
Limitations of Data:	The MHSIP Report Card Survey is in early stages of state implementation and the availability of data may differ across states. State surveys may be limited by numerous sources of error: e.g., coverage error, which is the result of neglecting to measure all parts of the population; nonresponse error, which is caused by individuals who refuse the survey or cannot be located; and sampling error, which reflects the difference between the general population and the specific sample chosen for the survey.

Measure Type:	Mental health consumer satisfaction outcome
Measure:	Percentage of persons (aged 18 and older) or their family members or both who are satisfied with: (a) access to mental health services, (b) appropriateness of services, and (c) perceptions of gain in personal outcomes.
Numerator:	All adults or family members of adults who are surveyed or both and are satisfied with access to and appropriateness of mental health services and gain in personal outcomes.
Denominator:	All adults or family members surveyed or both who use mental health services.
Rationale for Measure:	Satisfaction of the person using mental health services is a critical measure of the viability of service programs. If consumers are not satisfied with services, they may not use them.
Limitations of Measure:	Variations in consumer satisfaction surveys across states make interstate comparisons problematic.
Use of Measure:	This outcome measure should be used in conjunction with relevant process and capacity measures in order to gain a sense of whether the actions taken by the state agencies are having the desired impact.
Data Resources:	MHSIP Report Card Survey; state surveys.
Limitations of Data:	The MHSIP Report Card Survey is in early stages of implementation; the availability of the data may differ by states. State surveys may be limited by numerous sources of error: e.g., coverage error, which is the result of neglecting to measure all parts of the population; non-response error, which is caused by individuals who refuse the survey or cannot be located; and sampling error, which reflects the difference between the general population and the specific sample chosen for the survey.

Measure Type:	**Immunization health status outcome**
Measure:	**Reported incidence rate of representative vaccine-preventable diseases.**

Numerator:	Number of reported cases (for each disease, age, or risk group).
Denominator:	Population estimate (for each age or risk group).
Rationale for Measure:	Key objective used by CDC, states, and *Healthy People 2000*. (This measure corresponds to *Healthy People 2000* Objective 20.1.)
Limitations of Measure:	Incomplete coverage of population.
Use of Measure:	This outcome measure should be used in conjunction with relevant process and capacity measures in order to gain a sense of whether the actions taken by the state health agencies are having the desired impact.
Data Resources:	
Numerator:	State-based reportable disease registries.
Denominator:	Official state population estimate.
Limitations of Data:	Inconsistent validity and reliability; subject to selection and reporting bias; only some vaccine-preventable diseases are reported.

Measure Type:	Immunization risk status
Measure:	Age-appropriate vaccination rates for target age groups (children aged 2 years; children entering school at approximately 5 years of age; and adults aged 65 and older) for each major vaccine group.

Numerator:	Number of people within each age group who are appropriately vaccinated.
Denominator:	Population estimate for each age group.
Rationale for Measure:	Used by CDC and states to monitor health status and best measure of achievement of immuniza- tion objectives. (This measure corresponds to *Healthy People 2000* Objective 20.11.)
Limitations of Measure:	Incomplete coverage of population: does not include high-risk non-elderly adults or children aged 3-5 or high-risk subgroups (poor, under- served minorities, adolescents).
Use of Measure:	This outcome measure should be used in con- junction with relevant process and capacity measures in order to gain a sense of whether the actions taken by the state health agencies are having the desired impact.
Data Resources:	National Immunization Survey (NIS); retrospec- tive school-based surveys; Medicare Statistical System; HEDIS managed care data; BRFSS.
Limitations of Data:	Only a small percentage of NIS immunization histories are confirmed, although many states have the ability to confirm most of them. Medi- care data excludes those immunized in hospitals and HMOs, although HEDIS 3.0 calls for report- ing on influenza immunizations for Medicare recipients.

Measure Type:	Substance abuse health status outcome
Measure:	Death rate of persons aged 15-65 attributed to (a) alcohol, (b) other drug use, and (c) combined agents.

Numerator:	Number of alcohol and other drug-related deaths.
Denominator:	Number of deaths of persons between 15 and 65 years of age.
Rationale for Measure:	Alcohol and other drug use contribute to a wide variety of deaths, including fatal accidents. (This measure corresponds to *Healthy People 2000* Objective 4.1.)
Limitations of Measure:	Many personal and social factors can influence alcohol and drug use that are difficult for a state agency to measure in the short term. Traffic and highway drunk driving deaths may be affected by state and local enforcement of drunk driving laws. Some deaths may not occur for many years after use (e.g., cirrhosis).
Use of Measure:	This outcome measure should be used in conjunction with relevant process and capacity measures in order to gain a sense of whether the actions taken by the state agencies are having the desired impact.
Data Resources:	Death records in National Vital Statistics Systems; Fatal Accident Reporting System; traffic fatality reports; Mortality, Multiple Cause of Death Data.
Limitations of Data:	Cause of death is not always accurately reported and may be collected differently in different states.

Measure Type:	Substance abuse health status outcome
Measure:	Percentage of emergency room encounters for alcohol or other drug-related causes.

Numerator:	Number of encounters that mention alcohol or other drugs.
Denominator:	Total emergency room encounters.
Rationale for Measure:	Emergency room encounters are good indicators of heavy alcohol and illicit drug use.
Limitations of Measure:	The causes reported for emergency room encounters may understate the actual number of emergency room encounters due to alcohol or other drugs.
Use of Measure:	This outcome measure should be used in conjunction with relevant process and capacity measures in order to gain a sense of whether the actions taken by the state agencies are having the desired impact.
Data Resources:	Drug Abuse Warning Network; state emergency room data; hospital discharge data; Medicaid hospital and claims data.
Limitations of Data:	DAWN data are only available for selected hospitals within a state; therefore, statewide estimates will not be available from this source. A further complication may occur as managed care and medical facility consolidation progress, if the base of reporting systems of emergency room facilities deteriorates. Such erosion of the reporting base would cast doubt on the validity and reliability of performance demonstrated, even for a substate area, through the use of DAWN data or through Medicaid hospitalization data.

Measure Type:	**Substance abuse social functioning**
Measure:	**Prevalence rate of substance abuse clients who report experiencing diminished severity of problems after completing treatment as measured by the Addiction Severity Index (ASI) or a similar measure.**

Numerator:	Number of clients with reduced severity scores on given dimension.
Denominator:	Number of clients followed up after treatment.
Rationale for Measure:	Changes in the areas measured by the ASI (medical problems; employment or financial problems; alcohol and drug use; illegal activity; family or social problems; and psychological problems) are key indicators of treatment effectiveness.
Limitations of Measure:	Many personal and socioeconomic factors can influence alcohol and drug use that are difficult for a state agency to measure in the short term.
Use of Measure:	This outcome measure should be used in conjunction with relevant process and capacity measures in order to gain a sense of whether the actions taken by the state agencies are having the desired impact.
Data Resources:	Treatment Episode Data Set (if discharge and follow-up added); state client data systems (e.g., California Alcohol and Drug Data System, Iowa Substance Abuse Reporting System and Minnesota Treatment Accountability Program).
Limitations of Data:	Not all states collect ASI data because of cost considerations. Not all clients can be located for follow-up; follow-up periods may vary in different states; some states collect data on all clients, not just those paid for with block grant funds, making cross state comparisons misleading.

Measure Type:	Substance abuse social functioning
Measure:	Ratio of substance abuse clients involved with the criminal justice system before and after completing treatment.

Numerator:	Percentage of clients with arrests or convictions after completing treatment.
Denominator:	Percentage of clients with arrests or convictions before treatment.
Rationale for Measure:	Reduced crime (and the cost associated with it) is a key indicator of treatment effectiveness, especially for other drug users.
Limitations of Measure:	Criminal behavior can be affected by many factors that are not under the direct control of the state substance abuse agency, which typically does not have responsibility for delivering or administering services to jail or prison populations.
Use of Measure:	This outcome measure should be used in conjunction with relevant process and capacity measures in order to gain a sense of whether the actions taken by the state health agencies are having the desired impact.
Data Resources:	Uniform Crime Reporting; state client data systems (e.g., Colorado Drug/Alcohol Coordinated Data Systems).
Limitations of Data:	Not all clients can be located at follow-up; difficult to combine data from separate systems due to data privacy and other technical issues. State surveys may be limited by numerous sources of error: e.g., coverage error, which is the result of neglecting to measure all parts of the population; nonresponse error, which is caused by individuals who refuse the survey or cannot be located; and sampling error, which reflects the difference between the general population and the specific sample chosen for the survey.

Measure Type:	**Substance abuse risk status**
Measure:	**Prevalence rate of adolescents aged 14-17 engaged in heavy drinking* or other drug use.**

Numerator:	Number of adolescents who report heavy drinking* or using other drugs.
Denominator:	Number of adolescents.
Rationale for Measure:	Heavy drinking and other drug use can lead to severe consequences, such as driving accidents, sexual and other abuse, violence, and death. (This measure corresponds to *Healthy People 2000* Objectives 4.6 and 4.7.)
Limitations of Measure:	Many personal and socioeconomic factors can influence heavy drinking and drug use that are difficult for a state agency to influence in the short term. In addition, a school-based measure misses dropouts, who may be at increased risk for substance abuse.
Use of Measure:	This outcome measure should be used in conjunction with relevant process and capacity measures in order to gain a sense of whether the actions taken by the state agencies are having the desired impact.
Data Resources:	Youth Risk Behavior Surveillance System (YRBSS); state high school surveys.
Limitations of Data:	The methodology used to collect YRBSS data may vary significantly across states, making interstate comparisons with these data alone problematic. It should also be noted that the YRBSS is currently conducted in fewer than half of all states and often does not involve a representative sampling of schools in a given state.

---

*The most common definition of heavy drinking across states is five or more drinks on one occasion. If a state has defined heavy drinking to be other than five or more drinks, it could propose to use its definition in a performance agreement with the DHHS. Ultimately, it would be desirable for all states to use a common definition.

Measure Type:	**Substance abuse risk status**
Measure:	**Prevalence rate of persons aged 18 and older engaged in heavy drinking* or other drug use.**

Numerator:	Number of people aged 18 and older engaged in frequent heavy drinking* or other drug use.
Denominator:	Number of people aged 18 and older.
Rationale for Measure:	High-risk alcohol and other drug use can lead to severe consequences, such as death or permanent disability (traumatic brain injury).
Limitations of Measure:	Many personal and socioeconomic factors can influence alcohol and drug use that are difficult for a state agency to measure in the short term.
Use of Measure:	This outcome measure should be used in conjunction with relevant process and capacity measures in order to gain a sense of whether the actions taken by the state agencies are having the desired impact.
Data Resources:	Behavioral Risk Factor Surveillance System (BRFSS); state needs assessment surveys
Limitations of Data:	The methodology used to collect BRFSS data may vary significantly across states, making interstate comparisons with these data alone problematic. BRFSS may also underestimate use because of respondents' reluctance to report use to an interviewer over the telephone or because of missing populations without phones (e.g., the homeless and those living in institutions).

*The most common definition of heavy drinking across states is five or more drinks on one occasion. If a state has defined heavy drinking to be other than five or more drinks, it could propose to use its definition in a performance agreement with the DHHS. Ultimately, it would be desirable for all states to use a common definition.

Measure Type:	**Substance abuse risk status**
Measure:	**Percentage of women who gave birth in the past year and reported using alcohol or other drugs during pregnancy.**

Numerator:	Number of pregnant women who gave birth in the past year and reported using alcohol or other drugs.
Denominator:	All women giving birth in the state.
Rationale for Measure:	The use of these substances during pregnancy can lead to adverse birth outcomes (e.g., fetal alcohol syndrome). (This measure corresponds to *Healthy People 2000* Objective 14.10.)
Limitations of Measure:	Alcohol and drug use by a state's pregnant female population can be affected by many factors, including exposure to advertising, that may not be under the direct control of state agencies.
Use of Measure:	This outcome measure should be used in conjunction with relevant process and capacity measures in order to gain a sense of whether the actions taken by the state agencies are having the desired impact.
Data Resources:	Birth records; Behavioral Risk Factor Surveillance System (BFRSS); adverse pregnancy outcome registry; maternal and child health case management records
Limitations of Data:	The methodology used to collect BRFSS may vary significantly across states, making interstate comparisons problematic, unless supported by other data sources, such as state screening and reporting systems or medical information systems. Sample sizes may not be sufficiently large to accurately identify rates of substance abuse among the subpopulation of pregnant women.

Measure Type:	Substance abuse risk status
Measure:	**Mean age at first use of "gateway" drugs (tobacco, marijuana, alcohol)**

Numerator:	Mean age of children and adolescents reporting first use of tobacco, marijuana or alcohol.
Denominator:	Number of children and adolescents.
Rationale for Measure:	Early use of these substances may be a precursor of more serious drug use or abuse.
Limitations of Measure:	Measure does not distinguish between those who use gateway drugs and subsequently go on to further use and those whose first use does not lead to any subsequent behavior.
Use of Measure:	This outcome measure should be used in conjunction with relevant process and capacity measures in order to gain a sense of whether the actions taken by the state agencies are having the desired impact.
Data Resources:	Youth Risk Behavior Surveillance System (YRBSS); state student surveys
Limitations of Data:	The methodology used to collect YRBSS data may vary significantly across states, making interstate comparisons with these data alone problematic. It should also be noted that the YRBSS is currently conducted in fewer than half of all states and often does not involve a representative sampling of schools in a given state.

Measure Type:	**Substance abuse risk status**
Measure:	**Percentage of adolescents aged 14-17 stating disapproval of marijuana use.**

Numerator:	Number of adolescents indicating disapproval of marijuana use.
Denominator:	Number of adolescents.
Rationale for Measure:	Peer disapproval of marijuana use is a strong protective factor; when the percentage of youth with this attitude is high, marijuana rates tend to be low. (This measure corresponds to *Healthy People 2000* Objective 4.9)
Limitations of Measure:	Indirect measures may understate actual use, as high-risk populations (dropouts, incarcerated adolescents) are often not included in surveys.
Use of Measure:	This outcome measure should be used in conjunction with relevant process and capacity measures in order to gain a sense of whether the actions taken by the state agencies are having the desired impact.
Data Resources:	State surveys.
Limitations of Data:	Surveys are not available in many states, and where available may be limited by numerous sources of error: e.g., coverage error, which is the result of neglecting to measure all parts of the population; nonresponse error, which is caused by individuals who refuse the survey or cannot be located; and sampling error, which reflects the difference between the general population and the specific sample chosen for the survey.

Measure Type:	Substance abuse risk status
Measure:	Percentage of adolescents aged 14-17 who report parents or guardians who communicate non-use expectations.

Numerator:	Number of adolescents who report that parents or guardians clearly communicate the expectations of non-use.
Denominator:	Number of adolescents.
Rationale for Measure:	Parental expectation for non-use by their children is a significant protective factor. When the percentage of parents or guardians who clearly communicate a non-use message is high, use rates tend to be low.
Limitations of Measure:	Indirect measures may understate actual use, as high-risk populations (dropouts, incarcerated adolescents) are often not included in surveys.
Use of Measure:	This outcome measure should be used in conjunction with relevant process and capacity measures in order to gain a sense of whether the actions taken by the state agencies are having the desired impact.
Data Resources:	State surveys.
Limitations of Data:	Surveys are not available in many states, and where available may be limited by numerous sources of error: e.g., coverage error, which is the result of neglecting to measure all parts of the population; nonresponse error, which is caused by individuals who refuse the survey or cannot be located; and sampling error, which reflects the difference between the general population and the specific sample chosen for the survey.

Measure Type:	**Substance abuse risk status**
Measure:	**Percentage of drug abuse clients who engage in risk behaviors related to HIV/AIDS after completing treatment plan.**
Numerator:	Number of clients engaging in needle sharing and unprotected sex after completing treatment plan.
Denominator:	Number of clients followed up after completing treatment plan.
Rationale for Measure:	Drug and alcohol abusers are at high risk for HIV/AIDS due to needle sharing and unprotected sex.
Limitations of Measure:	Many personal and socioeconomic factors can influence alcohol and drug use that are difficult for a state agency to measure in the short term.
Use of Measure:	This outcome measure should be used in conjunction with relevant process and capacity measures in order to gain a sense of whether the actions taken by the state agencies are having the desired impact.
Data Resources:	State client data systems (e.g., Minnesota Drug and Alcohol Abuse Normative Evaluation System).
Limitations of Data:	Most states do not collect these data; collecting data on sexual behaviors can be controversial. State surveys may be limited by numerous sources of error: e.g., coverage error, which is the result of neglecting to measure all parts of the population; nonresponse error, which is caused by individuals who refuse the survey or cannot be located; and sampling error, which reflects the difference between the general population and the specific sample chosen for the survey.

Measure Type:	**Sexual assault health status outcome**
Measure:	**Incidence rate of sexual assault reported by females.**

Numerator:	Total number of sexual assaults reported by females.
Denominator:	State female population.
Rationale for Measure:	This is the key sexual assault indicator currently available. (This measure corresponds to *Healthy People 2000* Objective 7.12.)
Limitations of Measure:	Sexual assault experienced by a state's female population can be affected by many factors, including state law enforcement, availability of special educational programs for young adolescents, availability of counseling services for offenders, and other factors that may not be under the direct control of the state's health agency. The rate of sexual assaults of males, particularly those in prison, is omitted by this measure.
Use of Measure:	This outcome measure should be used in conjunction with relevant process and capacity measures in order to gain a sense of whether the actions taken by the state health agency are having the desired impact.
Data Resources:	
Numerator:	Sexual assault victims service providers; FBI; state police; criminal justice data systems.
Denominator:	Official state population estimate.
Limitations of Data:	The reported rate of sexual assault is widely regarded as understating the actual incidence of sexual assault; however, this may not be a problem if the ratio of reported to unreported assault remains relatively stable.

Measure Type:	**Disability health status outcome**
Measure:	**Percentage of newborns with neural tube defects.**

Numerator:	Infants borth with neural tube defects.
Denominator:	Total births.
Rationale for Measure:	Neural tube defects are dramatically reduced by appropriate folic acid intake prior to conception. (This measure corresponds to *Healthy People 2000* Objective 14.17.)
Limitations of Measure:	Neural tube defects may be affected by other factors that are not under the direct control of the state health agencies.
Use of Measure:	This outcome measure should be used in conjunction with relevant process and capacity measures in order to gain a sense of whether the actions taken by the state health agencies are having the desired impact.
Data Resources:	
Numerator:	Birth records or adverse pregnancy outcome registries.
Denominator:	Birth records.
Limitations of Data:	Neural tube defects may not always be recorded by medical or hospital staff.

Measure Type:	Disability social functioning
Measure:	Percentage of persons aged 18-65 with disabilities who are in the workforce.

Numerator:	Number of people aged 18-65 with disabilities who are in the workforce.
Denominator:	Number of people aged 18-65 with disabilities.
Rationale for Measure:	One measurement of functionality for an individual with a disability is employment.
Limitations of Measure:	There may be individuals with certain disabilities for whom working is not possible.
Use of Measure:	This outcome measure should be used in conjunction with relevant process and capacity measures in order to gain a sense of whether the actions taken by the state health agencies are having the desired impact.
Data Resources:	Current Population Survey (CPS); National Health Interview Survey (NHIS).
Limitations of Data:	The CPS only provides state-level estimates for approximately ten states.

Measure Type:	**Disability risk status**
Measure:	**Percentage of children aged 6 or younger with blood lead greater than 10 micrograms per deciliter.***

Numerator:	Number of children less than 6 years of age with blood lead levels greater than 10 micrograms per deciliter.
Denominator:	Number of children less than six years of age in state.
Rationale for Measure:	Lead intoxication has been demonstrated to result in decreased intelligence and social functionality. (This measure corresponds to *Healthy People 2000* Objective 11.4.)
Limitations of Measure:	Lead intoxication in young children living in a state can be affected by many factors, such as the average age of the housing stock, that may not be under the direct control of the health agencies.
Use of Measure:	This outcome measure should be used in conjunction with relevant process and capacity measures in order to gain a sense of whether the actions taken by the state health agencies are having the desired impact.
Data Resources:	
Numerator:	Reports of children with lead greater than 10 micrograms per deciliter to state health agencies. (In most states physicians and clinical labs are required to report these results.)
Denominator:	Official state population estimate.
Limitations of Data:	Physicians and clinical labs may not always report each incident of high blood lead levels; not all at-risk children may be tested.

---

*The numerical value in this measure is the level that is generally regarded as appropriate by the medical community; it does not represent a level that has been independently determined or endorsed by the panel.

Measure Type:	**Disability risk status**
Measure:	**Percentage of women who gave birth during the past year and reported using alcohol, tobacco, or other drugs during pregnancy.**

Numerator:	Number of women who gave birth during the past year and reported using alcohol, tobacco, or other drugs during pregnancy.
Denominator:	All women giving birth in the state.
Rationale for Measure:	Alcohol, tobacco, and other drug use during pregnancy is a leading cause of birth defects that can result in disability of newborns and in later stages of life. (This measure corresponds to *Healthy People 2000* Objective 14.10.)
Limitations of Measure:	Alcohol, tobacco, and other drug use by a state's pregnant female population can be affected by many factors, including exposure to advertising, availability of vending machines, and other factors that may not be under the direct control of the health agencies.
Use of Measure:	This outcome measure should be used in conjunction with relevant process and capacity measures in order to gain a sense of whether the actions taken by the state health agencies are having the desired impact.
Data Resources:	Birth records; Behavioral Risk Factor Surveillance System (BFRSS); adverse pregnancy outcome registry; maternal and child health case management records.
Limitations of Data:	It is widely understood that birth record data may understate the actual use of alcohol, tobacco, and other drugs by pregnant women. Nevertheless, this should not be a problem in examining trends over time or making intrastate comparisons if the reporting bias is consistent from one time period to another across jurisdictions. The methodology used to collect BRFSS data may vary significantly across states, making interstate comparisons problematic. Sample sizes may not be sufficiently large to accurately identify rates of substance abuse among the subpopulation of pregnant women.

Measure Type:	**Emergency medical services health status outcome**
Measure:	**Percentage of persons who suffer out-of-hospital cardiac arrest who survive.**
Numerator:	Number of people discharged from hospitals following out-of-hospital cardiac arrest.
Denominator:	All cases of out-of-hospital cardiac arrest.
Rationale for Measures:	Cardiac arrests are a leading cause of death. Promptly provided emergency medical services can increase the likelihood of survival.
Limitations of Measure:	The rate of cardiac arrest survival of a state's population can be affected by many factors, including the average age of its population, the percentage of its elderly population living in rural areas, and the quality of care provided by its hospitals' emergency medical rooms. None of these factors is within the control of a local or regional emergency medical services system.
Use of Measure:	This outcome measure should be used in conjunction with relevant process and capacity measures in order to gain a sense of whether the actions taken by EMS providers are having the desired impact.
Data Resources:	State EMS data systems.
Limitations of Data:	EMS data systems may vary significantly across states, making interstate comparisons problematic.

APPENDIX
D

Analysis of Comments on Draft Report

In September and October of 1996 nearly 3,000 copies of the draft report, "Assessment of Performance Measures in Public Health," were distributed for public comment both by the Department of Health and Human Services (DHHS) and the National Research Council (NRC). They were sent to a wide range of individuals and institutions, including various state government health agencies and professional associations. Recipients were invited to send comments or suggestions on the draft report, by mail, fax, or electronic mail. A total of 110 organizations and individuals supplied the panel with comments on the draft report, which are listed in the second section of this appendix.

The panel benefited greatly from the thoughtful and constructive comments on the draft report and wishes to thank each of the people who took the time to prepare comments. As can be seen from the list, the majority of the respondents were from state health agencies, representing mental health, alcohol and substance abuse, emergency medical services, family services, and preventive health. Other comments came from groups representing special populations, e.g., children and Native Americans of all ages.

Each comment was logged in and coded to enable the panel to review them efficiently. Comments ranged from brief to extensive, with many offering helpful suggestions for improving the report in various subject areas. The vast majority of the respondents praised the panel for providing a valuable framework for considering performance measures in public health, substance abuse, and mental health. Many commented on the care and thoughtfulness that was evident in the draft report, which are discussed in the next section.

Substantive issues raised by the respondents fell into six broad categories.

SUBSTANTIVE ISSUES

Addition of Subpopulations in PPG Agreements. Several organizations urged the panel to take into consideration various subpopulations of interest for the measures contained in the draft report, e.g., children and adolescents, ethnic and racial minorities, and persons with multiple health conditions:

> The failure to demonstrate the importance of ethnicity as variables throughout the health outcomes measures needs to be visited by the panel.
>
> I specifically request that services to Native Americans be included in the performance measures.
>
> There are no dual diagnosis measures proposed and there should be at least some process or capacity measures suggested.
>
> Measure smoking among 18-24 years of age in addition to all adults 18+.
>
> Percentage of school children who eat five or more servings of fruits and vegetables daily.

The comments convinced the panel that additional measures for children and youth were needed in a number of health areas covered in the report, as this group is at high-risk in virtually all states. As explained in the report, however, other populations of special interest to state health agencies can vary greatly across states; therefore, states should be encouraged to specify their own subpopulations of interest and focus their PPG efforts accordingly. The panel expects that specific priority populations will be a central element of performance agreements between states and DHHS.

Modifications to Draft Measures. Several organizations urged the panel to take into consideration modifications to the measures contained in the draft report. The majority of such comments asked the panel to consider making particular measures more specific; other comments asked for more standardization of measures across the health areas addressed in the report. Examples of the first type of comment included:

> The outcome measures for Substance Abuse consistently refer to "alcohol and drug abuse." It is preferable to use the terminology "abuse of alcohol and other drugs."
>
> The EMS process measure "Percentage of trauma patients going to trauma centers" needs elaboration and revision. "Trauma centers" need some definition since not every hospital that may describe itself as a trauma center meets criteria.
>
> Change the proposed measure of "percentage of children with blood lead greater than 15 micrograms per deciliter" to "the percentage of children under six years of age with blood lead of 10 micrograms per deciliter or greater."

Many of the suggestions for modifying the specific wording of measures contained in the draft report were accepted by the panel. For example, "intravenous drug" was changed to "injection drug" and "communicable" disease was changed to "vaccine-preventable" disease. Other wording changes were made to add greater clarity or specificity to the measure descriptions and to make them consistent (whenever possible) across the health areas considered by the panel. In addition, limitations of both the measures and the cited data sources were explicitly acknowledged.

Additions to PPG Measures. Several organizations urged the panel to consider additional PPG measures. In reviewing these suggestions, the panel paid careful attention to whether a proposed measure was supported by a viable data source for state-level PPG purposes, as well as whether the measure could satisfy the panel's selection guidelines: (1) be aimed at specific objectives and results oriented; (2) be meaningful and understandable; (3) be supported by adequate data; and (4) be valid, reliable, and responsive. Unfortunately, there were more than three times as many measures suggested for which there is no data source than suggestions for which a data source was specified. Examples of measures without a data source included:

> Percentage of merchants selling tobacco products to minors (under 18).
> An outcome should be developed to assure that primary care providers either receive supplemental training in mental health services or use standardized screening tools for assessing the mental health status of primary care patients.
> Percentage of adults, aged 35-44 who have never lost a permanent tooth due to dental caries or periodontal disease.

Examples of suggestions for measures with a data source in at least one state included:

> Percentage of children with serious emotional disorders enrolled in school who are progressing academically and socially.
> Rate of survival from out of hospital cardiac arrest.
> Percentage of peers stating disapproval of marijuana use.

The panel accepted several of the suggestions. The report includes additional measures of outcome and risk reduction measures in several of the health areas examined by the panel, e.g., mental health, substance abuse, and STDs, HIV, and tuberculosis. The panel did not include some other well developed outcome measures either because they fell outside the scope of the panel's activities (such as dental health) or because they fell into the category of process or capacity measures, which are not offered as an all-inclusive listing but only provided as examples of many that states may want to use.

Revisions to PPG Measure Classification. A few organizations expressed disagreement with the panel's classification of measures into outcome, process, and capacity:

> I think the listing of outcomes on page 5 for chronic diseases includes a number of things (percentage of women receiving pap smears, for instance) which are actually processes; I would list them as such.
>
> Despite the designation of 47 measures as outcome measures, many of them are process measures.
>
> The draft report incorrectly classifies community changes as processes rather than outcomes.
>
> Most of the document appears to measure individual change. In the field of prevention we may address organizational practices, community development, and changes in attitude.

In response to these kinds of comments, the panel provides additional clarification about the definitions used; see Chapter 1.

Criticism of Draft Outcome Measures. A number of reviewers expressed concern that particular outcome measures suggested that their agency would be held accountable for health outcomes that are affected by multiple factors, many of which are outside their immediate programmatic control. In particular, a number of substance abuse and mental health agencies expressed disagreement over the panel's use of population-based measures to monitor their performance:

> We are very concerned that the majority of proposed substance abuse indicators involve population-based data. By contrast, we are very supportive of those measures which are focused on treated populations.
>
> We are concerned that only three of the eight proposed Substance Abuse Outcome Measures address the outcomes of substance abuse clients. The remaining five outcome measures address issues of substance abuse within broad populations that are, for the most part, not recipients of services funded through our Administration.
>
> We recommend that the Council more specifically identify potential confounding variables in measuring outcomes and guidelines for risk adjusting for them. Otherwise, the proposed outcome measures are likely to reach false conclusions about program effectiveness.
>
> The measures chosen tend to reflect the public health perspective. They emphasize goals for the general population rather than for the seriously and persistently mentally ill.

In several cases the panel was persuaded that a measure contained in the draft report was not the most appropriate measure for PPG purposes. In some cases, suggested outcome measures were substituted for ones contained in the draft report (e.g., the EMS measure concerning cardiac arrest survival was deemed more appropriate that the one concerning central nervous system injuries); in other cases, measures were revised.

Although the panel recognizes that the traditional perspective of most administrators of substance abuse and mental health agencies is to ensure adequate and appropriate treatment for their clients—in contrast to the traditional public health perspective, which assumes responsibility for an entire at-risk population—the panel concludes that some population-based measures are appropriate for performance agreements. The panel recognizes, however, that in many of the health areas covered in this report, such measures cannot be affected, in the short run, solely by the actions taken by a given state agency. But, when combined with related process and capacity measures that are under the direct control of a state agency, such measures can provide useful insights regarding the state's progress in meeting important goals. Over the long run (5-10 years), state agencies should be able to demonstrate their impact on improving the functioning of their target populations, including those at risk of suffering from substance abuse and mental health problems.

Data Availability and Comparability Issues. Several organizations urged the panel to take into consideration various data issues. Several people observed that the measures contained in the draft report were not consistent with similar measures in *Healthy People 2000* or other indicator systems (e.g., HEDIS). The panel has attempted to make the measures contained the revised report identical to those in other indicator systems whenever possible. However, there are two reasons for having measures in this report worded differently from similar measures in other indicator systems: (1) performance *measures* should not contain explicit numerical goals, although performance *agreements* between states and DHHS would be expected to contain specific targets; and (2) the measures parallel the language used in the major surveys used to support the measure, since the data for those surveys, in effect, define the measure.

In reviewing comments on data, the panel made a distinction between issues concerning data availability, data comparability, and other broad data issues including cost considerations and validity of data sources. Data availability concerns included:

> The data resources listed to measure vaccination for high risk groups will not be able to measure vaccination rates for children 2-5 years, adolescents, and high-risk non-elderly adults without substantial increase in the sample size and cost.
>
> There is currently no data available on the number of children and adolescents who receive mental health services and live in noncustodial living situations.
>
> It may also be problematic for states to collect and report the data which you request if the data source falls outside the control of the State Mental Health Authority or the State Substance Abuse Authority.

Targeting and tracking individuals with "mental illness" will be difficult to aggregate, and certainly will not be uniform within the state or nation. Each state has different parameters for tracking, recording mental health client data.

All states will need to develop similar mechanisms to capture the information needed, otherwise the information obtained will not be useful for nationwide or statewide application or planning.

The Behavioral Risk Factor Surveillance System (BRFSS) will offer limited comparability across states.

The measure descriptions now specify more completely the exact populations that can be supported by each of the listed data sources. More importantly, the report underscores the point that not every state is expected or required to adopt the potential measures. The panel's assumption is that if a state does not have the data system available for a measure, that measure would, by definition, not be part of its performance agreement with DHHS. In addition, some states may have their own systems that are better than those available in other states. In such cases, the state would be expected to use those data instead of data from the source(s) listed in the report.

Although many state administrators raised a concern about data availability for one or more of the draft outcome measures, the panel does not intend that all of the measures would be expected of every state. If the data needed to support a given measure are only available for a limited number of states, that performance measure could be used only for those states. That measure could be used to examine the progress made in a particular state, quite apart from any state-to-state comparisons.

ORGANIZATIONS AND INDIVIDUALS
THAT PROVIDED COMMENTS

Advocacy, Inc.
Alabama Department of Mental Health and Mental Retardation
Alaska Department of Health and Social Services
American Social Health Association
American Public Health Association
Anishnabek Community and Family Services
Arizona Department of Economic Security
Arizona Department of Health Services, Division of Behavioral Health Services
Arkansas Department of Health
Association of State and Territorial Chronic Disease Program Directors
Association of State and Territorial Dental Directors
Association of State and Territorial Disability Prevention Programs
Association of State and Territorial Health Officials
Association of Trauma Surgeons

Atlanta Project
Norma K. Bowyer
California Department of Health Services, Health and Welfare Agency
California Mental Health Planning Council
Center for Research in Ambulatory Health Care Administration
Centers for Disease Control and Prevention
Coalition for American Trauma Care
Community Family Planning Council, United Way of New York City
Community Health Care Association of New York State
Connecticut Department of Mental Health and Addiction Services
Connecticut Department of Public Health
Jean R. Cox
County of Los Angeles, Department of Health Services, Office of AIDS Programs and Policy
Shirley Datz-Johnson
Davis County Courthouse, Utah
Delaware Department of Services for Children, Youth and Their Families
Delaware Health and Social Services, Division of Alcoholism, Drug Abuse and Mental Health
Department of Health and Human Services, Office of the Secretary
Department of Health and Human Services, Office of Minority Health
East Coast Prevention Consortium
Georgia Department of Human Resources
Hawaii Department of Health, Emergency Medical Services Systems Branch
Hawaii Department of Health, Alcohol and Drug Abuse Division
Illinois Department of Mental Health and Developmental Disabilities
Illinois Department of Public Health
Indiana State Department of Health
Inter-Tribal Council of Michigan, Inc.
Iowa Department of Public Health
Cabinet for Health Services, Commonwealth of Kentucky
Legal Action Center
Samuel Lin, M.D., Ph.D.
Maryland Department of Health and Mental Hygiene, Alcohol and Drug Abuse Administration
Massachusetts Department of Public Health and Mental Health
Massachusetts Department of Public Health, Executive Office of Health and Human Services
Michigan Department of Community Health
Michigan Community Public Health Agency
Minnesota Department of Health
Minnesota Department of Human Services
Mississippi Department of Health

Mississippi Department of Mental Health
Missouri Department of Health
Missouri Department of Mental Health
Morrow & Morrow
National Alliance of Sexual Assault Coalitions
National Association of County & City Health Officials
National Association of State Alcohol and Drug Abuse Directors, Inc.
National Association of State Emergency Medical Services Directors
National Association of State Mental Health Program Directors
National Center for Health Statistics
National Coalition Against Sexual Assault
Nebraska Department of Health
New Jersey Department of Health and Senior Services
New Jersey Department of Human Services, Division of Mental Health and
    Hospitals
New Jersey Office of Emergency Medical Services
New Mexico Department of Health
New York State Department of Health
New York State Office of Alcoholism and Substance Abuse Services
New York State Office of Mental Health
North Carolina Department of Human Resources
North Carolina Department of Environment, Health and Natural Resources
North Dakota Department of Health
Ohio Department of Health
Oklahoma Department of Mental Health and Substance Abuse Services
Pennsylvania Department of Health
Project Rehab
L. James L. Rivers
Max Schneier
Science and Epidemiology Committee
Society for Public Health Education, Inc.
State Block Grant Coordinators
State EMS Directors Association
State of South Carolina
State Rape Prevention Program Directors
Substance Abuse and Mental Health Services Administration
Tennessee Department of Health
Texas Department of Health
Texas Department of Mental Health and Mental Retardation
United South and Eastern Tribes, Inc.
University of Alabama at Birmingham, School of Medicine
State of Utah
Utah Department of Health

Vermont Office of Alcohol and Drug Abuse Programs
Virginia Department of Health
Virginia Department of Mental Health, Mental Retardation and Substance Abuse Services
Virginia Mental Health Planning Council
Washington Department of Social and Health Services
Wisconsin Department of Health and Family Services
Wisconsin Department of Health and Social Services.